O A N L
OXFORD AMERICAN NEUROLOGY LIBRARY

Parkinson's Disease

O A N L
OXFORD AMERICAN NEUROLOGY LIBRARY

Parkinson's Disease

Edited by

Tanya Simuni, MD

Associate Professor of Neurology
Director, Parkinson's Disease and Movement Disorders Center
Northwestern University
Feinberg School of Medicine
Chicago, IL

Rajesh Pahwa, MD

Laverne and Joyce Rider Professor of Neurology
Director, Parkinson's Disease and Movement Disorder Center
University of Kansas Medical Center
Kansas City, KS

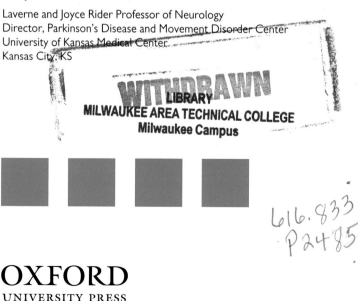

OXFORD
UNIVERSITY PRESS

OXFORD
UNIVERSITY PRESS

Oxford University Press, Inc., publishes works that further
Oxford University's objective of excellence
in research, scholarship, and education.

Oxford New York

Auckland Cape Town Dar es Salaam Hong Kong Karachi
Kuala Lumpur Madrid Melbourne Mexico City Nairobi
New Delhi Shanghai Taipei Toronto

With offices in
Argentina Austria Brazil Chile Czech Republic France Greece
Guatemala Hungary Italy Japan Poland Portugal Singapore
South Korea Switzerland Thailand Turkey Ukraine Vietnam

Copyright © 2009 by Oxford University Press, Inc.

Published by Oxford University Press, Inc.
198 Madison Avenue, New York, New York 10016
www.oup.com

Oxford is a registered trademark of Oxford University Press

Library of Congress Cataloging-in-Publication Data

Parkinson's disease / edited by Tanya Simuni, Rajesh Pahwa.
p. ; cm. — (Oxford American neurology library)
Includes bibliographical references.
ISBN 978-0-19-537172-7
1. Parkinson's disease.   I. Simuni, Tanya.   II. Pahwa, Rajesh.   III. Series.
[DNLM: 1. Parkinson Disease. WL 359 P24667 2008]
RC382.P243 2008
616.8'33—dc22   2008009497

9 8 7 6 5 4 3 2 1
Printed in the United States of America
on acid-free paper

Acknowledgment

We would like to express our gratitude to the National Parkinson Foundation for its support of and commitment to patient care.

Preface

Parkinson's disease (PD) is the second most common neurodegenerative disease after Alzheimer's disease. It currently afflicts a million people in the United States, and it is estimated that the prevalence of the disease will grow substantially with the aging of the population over the next two decades.

While the cause of PD remains unknown, there has been tremendous progress in the understanding of the pathophysiology of the disease and development of novel therapeutic strategies. Recent years have been marked by exponential growth in the number of pharmacological agents for PD, further development and refinement of surgical treatment options, and recognition of the importance of the nonmotor manifestations of PD.

This book was developed as a practical, up-to-date, concise guide for clinicians, and it aims to provide an overview of the spectrum of the clinical manifestations, etiology, diagnosis, and differential diagnosis of PD, with a focus on treatment interventions.

The editors thank all contributing authors for their expertise.

Contents

Contributors

Arif Dalvi, MD
University of Chicago
Chicago, IL

Hubert Fernandez, MD
University of Florida
McKnight Brain Institute
Gainesville, FL

Stewart Isaacson, MD
Parkinson's Disease and
Movement Disorders Center
Boca Raton, FL

Ioannis U. Isaias, MD
Mount Sinai Medical Center
New York, NY

Danna Jennings, MD
Institute for Neurodegenerative
Disorders
New Haven, CT

Benzi M. Kluger, MD
University of Florida
McKnight Brain Institute
Gainesville, FL

Kelly Lyons, PhD
University of Kansas Medical
Center
Kansas City, KS

Ariane Park, MD, MPH
Duke University Medical Center
Durham, North Carolina

Alex Rajput, MD
Division of Neurology
University of Saskatchewan
Saskatoon, Saskatchewan,
Canada

Indu Subramanian, MD
UCLA
Santa Monica, CA

Michele Tagliati, MD
Mount Sinai Medical Center
New York, NY

Aleks Videnovic, MD
Northwestern University
Feinberg School of Medicine
Chicago, IL

Ryan Walsh, MD, PhD
University of Chicago
Chicago, IL

Cindy Zadikoff, MD
Northwestern University
Feinberg School of Medicine
Chicago, IL

Chapter 1

Spectrum of clinical manifestations

Alex Rajput

Parkinson's disease (PD) was named for British physician James Parkinson (1755–1824), who described the condition in 1817 based on his observations of six persons in London, England, only three of whom he examined in person.

Epidemiology

Parkinson's disease is the second most common neurodegenerative condition in humans, after Alzheimer's disease. Studies have reported overall prevalence in the general population of between 84/100,000 and 775/100,000.[1] There is a clear increase in PD prevalence with age. A Dutch study reported prevalence of 1400/100,000 in those aged 55 to 64 years and 4300/100,000 in those aged 85 to 94 years.[2] In the institutionalized older population, the prevalence of PD has been estimated at 9% in one Canadian study,[3] with similar values in Australia.[4] PD affects at least 1% of the population aged 60 and older and 0.3% of the general population in the industrial world.[5] Studies in Europe and North America have yielded annual incidence rate estimates that range from 16 to 20 per 100,000.[6] The mean age of onset of PD is in the early 60s, but up to 10% of those with PD have onset prior to age 40. Onset at a young age does warrant consideration of other causes of parkinsonism. The majority of studies report a male predominance, with a roughly 3:2 ratio of males to females.[7] The lifetime risk for developing PD is reported as 4.4% for males and 3.7% for females.[8]

Economic burden

The cost of illness can be measured in direct (medications and health-care use) and indirect (lost productivity, cost of providing care, mortality) costs. In the United States, the increased direct medical care costs for PD patients amount to more than $10,000 annually compared with controls. The total annual health-care costs are almost $12,000 greater compared with controls. Almost 50% of the total economic cost of PD was due to lost productivity, with just under 20% each for inpatient care and uncompensated care; prescription drug costs accounted for less than 5% of the total cost. Combining direct and indirect costs, the annual cost of PD in the United States is nearly $23 billion. With the population aged 65 and older projected to be 80 million by 2040 in the United States, a conservative estimate of PD cost at that time is at least $50 billion annually (in 2002 dollars).[9]

Cardinal motor manifestations

The four cardinal features of PD are resting tremor, bradykinesia, rigidity, and postural instability. Presence of any two of the first three features is often used to make a clinical diagnosis of PD; the UK Brain Bank criteria, however, require a diagnosis of bradykinesia in conjunction with at least one additional feature.[10] Some use the mnemonic aid TRAP, which represents tremor, rigidity, akinesia (bradykinesia), and postural instability. As postural instability is usually not an early feature of PD and is a common finding in the elderly, a number of clinicians do not use this as a diagnostic feature. Another way to think of the cardinal features of PD is the so-called three S's: slow (bradykinesia), stiff (rigidity), and shaky (resting tremor) (Table 1.1).

Asymmetry is also common with PD, and in general the side that is affected earliest is the worst.

Dopamine, the key neurotransmitter involved in PD, is made by neurons in the substantia nigra and transported to the striatum (caudate and putamen) via the nigrostriatal pathway. The substantia nigra, caudate, and putamen are part of the extrapyramidal system. An adequate amount of dopamine in the extrapyramidal system is required for optimal functioning of the pyramidal (corticospinal) system. Approximately 50% striatal dopamine loss is needed before clinical features of PD appear, with an estimated preclinical period of about 6 years.

The diagnosis of PD is clinical and there are no readily available laboratory tests to confirm or refute the diagnosis. Definite diagnosis of PD is confirmed at autopsy, with neuronal loss and Lewy body inclusions in the substantia nigra and other brain stem nuclei.

Bradykinesia

Bradykinesia means, literally, slow movements. The term may also be used to encompass hypokinesia (diminished amplitude of movements),

Table 1.1 Cardinal features of Parkinson's disease (the 3 S's)
Slow (bradykinesia)
Stiff (rigidity)
Shaky (resting tremor)
Two of three are required to make the diagnosis
Onset is typically asymmetrical
Postural instability seen later in disease

bradykinesia (slow movements), and akinesia (absence of movement). Bradykinesia correlates best with dopamine loss in the striatum (particularly the putamen) and responds well to the cardinal features of dopaminergic replacement.

A patient's history may include reports of generalized slowness or difficulty with specific tasks, particularly fine motor skills such as fastening buttons and typing. One leg may drag and the ipsilateral arm swing may be reduced. Other typical manifestations include slower, more deliberate movements; smaller (micrographic) handwriting; and softer (hypophonic) speech.

Patients often complain of feeling "weak," yet PD does not cause muscle weakness on manual strength testing. Rather, patients are unable to generate force quickly enough to swing a golf club or open a jar easily. Motor sequencing of complex movements is impaired in PD. Interestingly, in times of stress, such as when a fire alarm goes off, the PD patient can move surprisingly fast, a reaction that is called *kinesia paradoxica*. This implies that the underlying motor programs are preserved in PD but are not accessed properly.

Testing for bradykinesia in the upper limbs includes tapping the index finger against the thumb, opening and closing the fingers, or alternating pronation/supination of the forearms (with a "turning a doorknob" motion). A handwriting sample should be obtained, and the patient should be asked if it looks different than usual. Testing in the lower limbs includes the task of foot tapping. The patient should be asked to cock the foot up (dorsiflex), bring the heel three inches off the ground, and tap the heel on the ground. One should observe for slowness, hesitation, and fatiguing of movements.

Rigidity

Rigidity is defined as increased tone detected on physical examination that is independent of speed and direction of movement. It is seen with diseases of the basal ganglia (extrapyramidal system) and is one of the cardinal features of PD. Spasticity, on the other hand, is increased tone that is dependent on both the speed and direction of movement and is present with lesions of the corticospinal or pyramidal tract system that occurs in stroke or multiple sclerosis.

The most common form of rigidity is known as cogwheeling—a ratchety sensation with passive movement at a joint. There is another type of rigidity called "lead pipe," a uniformly increased resistance to passive movement. The latter is analogous to the sensation of bending a spoon when trying to scoop out ice cream that is frozen too hard to be scooped easily.

Rigidity is tested by passive movement at a joint, typically the wrist, with the examiner moving the joint unpredictably in all directions. It is more easily brought out by having the patient tap the contralateral foot up and down or perform mental arithmetic (facilitation maneuver). If the patient has significant resting tremor at the wrist, it is better to test at the elbow. In the lower limb, one can test at the knee or the ankle. Similar to bradykinesia, rigidity responds quite well to dopaminergic therapy.

Tremor

Resting tremor is the most obvious feature of PD. The classic parkinsonian tremor is a "pill rolling" tremor at 4 to 6 Hz. Initially the tremor may be intermittent, typically affecting only one limb or even just a finger before becoming more constant. Tremor affecting the upper limb is often noted when the limb is at rest but disappears (or markedly improves) when the limb is active, such as when using a screwdriver or holding a cup. Evaluation of resting tremor should include examination with the limb fully supported against gravity (i.e., lying supine). While standing, there may be asymmetric tremor of the upper limbs. Other sites of tremor include the lips, chin, and legs. Head or voice tremors are uncommon in PD and should raise suspicion of essential type tremor.

The anatomic site responsible for tremor in PD is not well established, though the ventral intermediate nucleus of the thalamus is believed to be involved, as brain surgery with thalamotomy or deep brain stimulation improves the tremor in PD.[11] There is poor correlation with nigrostriatal dopamine deficiency and tremor. Severe tremor is often less responsive to medical therapy than bradykinesia and rigidity are.

Gait and posture

Gait and postural abnormalities (Table 1.2) are very common in PD. Early in the disease, only reduced unilateral arm swing may be evident. As the disease progresses there may be dragging of one leg, flexed posture, and a slow, shuffling gait. Later, patients develop gait initiation hesitation and difficulty in changing direction of gait. Patients may use so-called en bloc turning, in which several small steps are required to change direction rather than pivoting on one foot. PD patients may have difficulty getting in and out of a chair or bed. In particular, difficulty is greatest with low, soft chairs without armrests. Other terms used to describe PD gait are propulsion and retropulsion. Propulsion is a progressive running forward caused by a combination of stooped posture (which results in forward displacement of the body's center of gravity) and difficulty with gait initiation. In retropulsion, the patient takes several uncontrolled steps backward. The latter typically occurs after the patient first stands up. Both propulsion and retropulsion often result in falls.

Postural instability is usually a sign of late PD; however, it is common in older patients and is often multifactorial. In order to test for postural instability, the practitioner should stand behind the patient. The patient's feet should be shoulder-width apart. After explaining that the patient will be pulled backward, the practitioner should pull the patient backward, giving a moderate tug at the shoulders. *The patient should always be pulled, never pushed.* One step backward is acceptable; two to three steps is borderline, and four or more steps or loss of balance indicates the posture is unstable. If the posture is unstable, the test should be repeated to make certain that the patient was not simply caught off guard. In some cases patients make no attempt to correct their balance and would fall backward like a pole if not caught. The individual performing the test should *always* make sure to be prepared to catch the patient. *If need be, the tester should stand against a wall for support.*

Gait freezing

The anatomic site responsible for gait freezing is not well understood. Gait freezing most often occurs when the patient changes direction or crosses a threshold, such as when stepping into an elevator or going through a doorway. Placement of visual cues at such sites, such as strips of masking tape on the floor, may be enough to help the patient overcome gait freezing. An individual's inability to walk upon first standing up is referred to as *gait initiation failure* and is essentially the same as gait freezing. Gait freezing is seen in more advanced cases and can lead to falls. Unfortunately, gait freezing responds poorly to medical therapy.

Motor symptoms as complications of dopaminergic therapy

Dyskinesia means, literally, abnormal movements. These are involuntary movements, often choreiform and sometimes dystonic. They appear as fidgety, writhing movements and can affect the limbs, face, and truncal musculature. These movements are secondary to medical treatment of PD, most commonly due to levodopa. The cardinal features of PD may be minimal or absent when the patient is dyskinetic.

The *wearing off* of medication is a predictable loss of benefit that occurs prior to a patient's next dosage. For example, the patient experiences worsened tremor and slowness a half-hour before his scheduled dosage. This is most commonly seen with levodopa therapy. In general, wearing off does not appear early in the course of treatment but becomes more prevalent after a few years. In contrast to dyskinesias, which for some patients are mild and not bothersome, patients tend to be quite troubled by wearing off. Dyskinesias and wearing off are discussed further in Chapter 7.

Caveats

Musculoskeletal problems and pain can interfere with interpretation of physical findings. Previous strokes can cause increased tone (typically spasticity) and slowness. In older patients, mild parkinsonian signs (bradykinesia, rigidity, and gait/postural changes) are not uncommon and are much more frequent in those with dementia. Resting tremor, however, should not be considered a "normal" sign of aging.

Essential tremor

Essential tremor (ET) is reported to be 10 times as common as PD and may affect persons of any age, including children. There is often a family history of tremor. ET causes action and/or postural tremor in the upper limbs. The tremor disappears or markedly improves with rest. There may be associated head or voice tremor. As it is an action tremor, the tremor is much more debilitating than tremor in PD. There is no bradykinesia or rigidity in ET (see Chapter 3 for further details).

Features not typical of PD

It is important to note that early symptoms of falls, dementia, significant autonomic dysfunction, and hallucinations are not typical for PD. Ataxia,

Table 1.2 Supportive features of Parkinson's disease
Gait
• Reduced arm swing (asymmetric)
• Flexed posture
• Shuffling gait
• Slow to change directions (en bloc turning)
• Gait freezing
Unstable posture (not typical early in disease)
Hypophonia (softer voice)
Hypomimia (reduced facial expression)
Micrographia (smaller and slower writing)

hyper-reflexia, impaired eye movements, and persistent marked asymmetry of findings are also not seen in PD as a rule. See Chapter 3 for the differential diagnosis with criteria for atypical parkinsonian syndromes.

Spectrum of nonmotor manifestations

While the diagnosis of PD is based on the presence of cardinal motor signs, there are also many associated nonmotor features (Table 1.3). This aspect of PD is gaining increased recognition, although it is still underappreciated. Nonmotor features are generally not identified by more than half of neurological consultations for PD, and sleep disturbance has been unrecognized in more than 40% of cases.[12] The nonmotor symptoms of PD can be more disabling and cause more impact on disease-related quality of life impairment than the motor symptoms.[13] A screening questionnaire has been developed to identify nonmotor symptoms. Management of nonmotor PD features are discussed in Chapter 8.

Neuropsychiatric/behavioral disorders

Depression is the most common neuropsychiatric manifestation of PD. Mood dysfunction is not simply a reaction to developing PD, as depression can precede onset of PD's motor manifestations. A retrospective study showed that the risk of subsequent PD is 3 times greater in depressed individuals than in those who are not diagnosed with depression.[14] The reported prevalence of depression in PD ranges from 4% to 76%.[15,16] The wide variation in this range is attributed to inconsistency in study methodologies, choice of diagnostic instrument, and the definition of depression, as the profile of PD-associated depression may be different from that of patients with idiopathic depression. PD patients with depression generally have lower levels of guilt; feelings of self-reproach or failure; and higher levels of anxiety, pessimism, irrationality, and suicidal ideation than patients with primary depression.[17] The high rate of anxiety, which is present in up to 40% of patients, makes it the second most common affective disorder in PD. Apathy and social withdrawal are also more common in PD than in idiopathic depression. Anhedonia, or loss of interest in activities that previously were enjoyed, can be a common manifestation of PD. The intensity of mood dysfunction in PD can correlate with motor fluctuations.

Dementia was not initially thought to be a feature of PD. Despite the obvious motor findings, James Parkinson described PD with "the senses and intellects being uninjured." Dementia is uncommon in early PD, though careful neuropsychological testing reveals mild deficits in up to one-third of patients at the time of diagnosis (executive dysfunction and impairment of free recall with intact cognition and cued recall).[18] The overall prevalence of dementia in PD is estimated at between 20% and 40%, with relative risk of developing dementia nearly 6 times greater than in age-matched controls. A worse outcome is seen in demented PD patients, with greater risk of hip fractures and nursing home placement.[19] PD subjects with postural instability and gait difficulty are reported to be at greater risk of developing dementia.[20]

Hallucinations in PD are predominantly (though not exclusively) due to medical therapy. Dementia and cognitive impairment are risk factors for hallucinations, while age, duration, and severity of disease are inconsistently associated with hallucinations. Hallucinations occur in 30% of medically treated PD patients. Nonthreatening visual hallucinations (such as animals or small children) are the most common. Insight as a rule is preserved, though older demented individuals can become confused and delusional. All medications used to treat PD may cause hallucinations, though it is most commonly linked to the dopamine agonists, amantadine, and levodopa.

Behaviors associated with lack of impulse control, including compulsive gambling, shopping, pathological sexual behavior, and binge eating, are more common with PD than in the general population. Compulsive self-medication with dopaminergic drugs and punding (stereotypical non-purposeful behavior, such as sorting or lining up objects) are also reported with PD. The pathophysiology is not well defined but is thought to be related to dysfunction of the mesolimbic dopaminergic system, which is involved with behavior and motivation. The lifetime prevalence of compulsive shopping, pathological sexual behavior, and compulsive gambling combined is reported at 6.1%, and at 13.7% in PD patients on dopamine agonists.[21] The effect of dopamine agonists is a class effect and not specific to one drug or type of agonist, and may occur irrespective of dose. Levodopa use increases the risk of the reward-seeking and repetitive behaviors, but less so compared to the dopamine agonists. The lifetime prevalence of gambling alone in PD is 3.4%, and up to 7.2% for PD patients on agonists. Both values are significantly higher than the 1% lifetime prevalence of pathological gambling in the general population.[21] Patients and families should be cautioned about the increased risk of lack of impulse control before starting dopamine agonist therapy.

Sleep disorders

Sleep is frequently disrupted in PD patients. Reported prevalence rates of sleep disorders range from 75% to 98% in PD patients.[22,23] Sleep disorders in PD can be classified into three general categories: (1) disorders of sleep initiation and maintenance, (2) parasomnias, and (3) excessive daytime sleepiness (EDS). The reasons are multiple and include PD-related motor disability, nocturia, medication effects, and neuropathological changes affecting the structures responsible for the control of the sleep-wake cycle. An in-depth discussion of sleep dysfunction in PD is beyond the scope of this chapter, but the more common manifestations are briefly reviewed below.

Rapid eye movement (REM) behavior disorder is caused by a loss of the muscle atonia that normally occurs in REM sleep. Individuals with REM behavior disorder may literally "act out" their dreams with punching, kicking, and shouting and in some cases may injure themselves or their bed partner. REM behavior disorder occurs in about one-third of PD cases, and REM behavior disorder may precede PD in up to 40% of cases.[24]

Restless legs syndrome (RLS) affects up to 5% of the general population and 10% of those aged 65 years and older.[25] Among PD patients, nearly 20% have RLS, and in more than 70% of those with PD and RLS, the PD symptoms precede the RLS.[26]

Excessive daytime sleepiness (EDS) occurs in nearly half of patients with PD.[24] Sudden onset of sleepiness, or so-called sleep attacks, may occur in 1% of patients with PD. A high score on the Epworth Sleepiness Scale, increased PD duration, and treatment with dopamine agonists were risk factors.[27] Physicians should be vigilant about screening for EDS and counsel the patient regarding the risk of EDS with initiation of dopaminergic therapy.

Gastrointestinal and genitourinary disorders

Constipation is common in PD. In the Honolulu-Asia Aging Study, a longitudinal study of aging in men, reduced frequency of bowel movements portended a greater risk of developing PD.[28]

Dysphagia is common in PD but usually occurs in advanced stages of the disease. There is a disparity between radiologically detected dysphagia and clinically symptomatic dysphagia, with the former far in excess of the latter. Excess saliva is due to reduced spontaneous swallowing, not to overproduction of saliva. The severity can range from mild nocturnal drooling to constant daytime drooling, which is socially embarrassing and affects oral health.

Increased urinary frequency and urgency are common. Normally, the basal ganglia exert an inhibitory effect on the pontine micturition center, allowing the bladder to be "quiet" during filling. In PD this inhibitory effect is lost and the bladder becomes hyperactive. Urge incontinence may result, particularly if the patient cannot mobilize quickly enough to get to a bathroom. In males, an enlarged prostate can cause urinary frequency and should not be ignored as a potential cause of bladder symptoms. Impaired sexual function is more common in PD than in age-matched controls and is most likely multifactorial in nature.

Orthostatic hypotension

Symptoms of prominent orthostasis are usually associated with the advanced stages of PD and are partially attributed to the hypotensive effect of dopaminergic therapy. However, orthostasis can be an early manifestation of PD and does not always signify an alternative etiology of parkinsonism, such as multiple system atrophy.

Sensory

Some PD patients complain of pain. Usually it is an aching pain in the limb or limbs that are most severely affected. Painful early morning dystonia typically affects the lower limbs and improves after medication. Pain may be a feature of wearing off. Other causes of pain that should be considered are pain from a fall, arthritis, muscle strain, and so on. Painful stiff shoulder and restricted range of motion in the more affected limb can be an early manifestation of PD leading to orthopedic evaluations prior to PD diagnosis. Tingling and numbness are occasionally reported by PD patients.

Olfactory dysfunction in PD is well known and may precede onset of motor symptoms by several years. Pathologically, the olfactory bulb system is affected before loss of neurons in the substantia nigra causes motor findings.

Visual dysfunction, which is often reported in PD, may simply be blurred vision or "tired eyes" when reading. Well-documented abnormalities in PD include convergence insufficiency, abnormal color discrimination, and impaired visual contrast sensitivity. Slight reduction in visual acuity has also been reported in PD. Dopamine is found throughout the visual pathway, and retinal dopamine deficiency has the strongest link to visual dysfunction in PD, particularly for color vision.

Other nonmotor manifestations

The pathophysiology of fatigue in PD is not well understood. Some patients note improvement in fatigue following medical treatment. Seborrheic dermatitis is more common in patients with PD, and typically affects the face and scalp.

Table 1.3 Nonmotor features associated with Parkinson's disease
Neuropsychiatric/behavioral
• Depression
• Dementia
• Apathy
• Hallucinations
• Impulse-control disorders
Sleep disorders
• Insomnia
• Hypersomnolence
• REM behavior disorder
• Restless legs syndrome

Table 1.3 *continued*

Gastrointestinal, genitourinary, and autonomic dysfunction

- Constipation
- Dysphagia
- Drooling
- Urinary urgency
- Sexual dysfunction
- Orthostatic hypotension

Sensory

- Pain, paresthesias
- Olfactory dysfunction
- Visual dysfunction

Other

- Fatigue
- Seborrhea

Summary

PD is the second most common neurodegenerative condition affecting humans. While the diagnosis of PD is based on the presence of cardinal manifestations of motor disability, recent literature has highlighted the significance of nonmotor features of PD that for some patients are more disabling than the motor manifestations.

References

1. Rajput M, Rajput A, Rajput AH. Epidemiology. In: Pahwa R, Lyons K, eds. *Handbook of Parkinson's Disease.* 4th ed. New York: Informa Healthcare; 2007:19–27.

2. de Rijk MC, Breteler MMB, Graveland GA, et al. Prevalence of Parkinson's disease in the elderly: the Rotterdam study. *Neurology.* 1995;45:2143–2146.

3. Moghal S, Rajput AH, Meleth R, D'Arcy C, Rajput R. Prevalence of movement disorders in institutionalized elderly. *Neuroepidemiology.* 1995;14:297–300.

4. Chan DK, Dunne M, Wong A, Hu E, Hung WT, Beran RG. Pilot study of prevalence of Parkinson's disease in Australia. *Neuroepidemiology.* 2001;20:112–117.

5. de Lau LML, Breteler MMB. Epidemiology of Parkinson's disease. *Lancet Neurol.* 2006;5:525–535.

6. Twelves D, Perkins KSM, Counsell C. Systematic review of incidence studies of Parkinson's disease. *Mov Disord.* 2003;18:19–31.

7. Schrag A, Ben-Schlomo Y, Quinn N. How valid is the clinical diagnosis of Parkinson's disease in the community? *J Neurol Neurosurg Psych.* 2002; 73:529–535.

8. Elbaz A, Bower JH, Maraganore DM, et al. Risk tables for parkinsonism and Parkinson's disease. *J Clin Epidemiol.* 2002;55:25–31.

9. Huse DM, Schulman K, Orsini L, Castelli-Haley J, Kennedy S, Lenhart G. Burden of illness in Parkinson's disease. *Mov Disord.* 2005;20(11):1449–1454.

10. Hughes AJ, Daniel SE, Kilford L, Lees AJ. Accuracy of clinical diagnosis of idiopathic Parkinson's disease: a clinico-pathological study of 100 cases. *J Neurol Neurosurg Psychiatry*. 1992;55:181–184.

11. Chou KL, Hurtig HI. Classical motor features of Parkinson's disease. In: Pfeiffer RF, Bodis-Wollner I, eds. *Parkinson's Disease and Nonmotor Dysfunction*. New York: Humana Press; 2005:171–181.

12. Chaudhuri KR, Martinez-Martin P, Schapira AHV, et al. International multicenter pilot study of the first comprehensive self-completed nonmotor symptoms questionnaire for Parkinson's disease: the NMSQuest study. *Mov Disord*. 2006;21:916–923.

13. The Global Parkinson's Disease Survey (GPDS) Steering Committee. Factors impacting on quality of life in Parkinson's disease: results from an international survey. *Mov Disord*. 2002;17:60–67.

14. Schuurman AG, van den Akker M, Ensinck KT, et al. Increased risk of Parkinson's disease after depression: a retrospective cohort study. *Neurology*. 2002;58:1501–1504.

15. McDonald WM, Richard IH, DeLong MR. Prevalence, etiology, and treatment of depression in Parkinson's disease. *Biol Psychiatry*. 2003;54:363–375.

16. Veazey C, Aki SO, Cook KF, Lai EC, Kunik ME. Prevalence and treatment of depression in Parkinson's disease. *J Neuropsychiatry Clin Neurosci*. 2005;17:310–323.

17. Cummings JL. Depression and Parkinson's disease: a review. *Am J Psychiatry*. 1992;149:443–454.

18. Troster AI, Woods SP. Neuropsychological aspects. In: Pahwa R, Lyons KE, eds. *Handbook of Parkinson's Disease*. 4th edition. New York: Informa Healthcare; 2007:109–131.

19. Kavanagh P, Marder K. Dementia. In: Pfeiffer RF, Bodis-Wollner I, eds. *Parkinson's Disease and Nonmotor Dysfunction*. New York: Humana Press; 2005:35–47.

20. Alves G, Larsen JP, Emre M, Wentzel-Larsen T, Aarsland D. Changes in motor subtype and risk for incident dementia in Parkinson's disease. *Mov Disord*. 2006;21:1123–1130.

21. Voon V, Hassan K, Zurowski M, et al. Prevalence of repetitive and reward-seeking behaviors in Parkinson disease. *Neurology*. 2006;67:1254–1257.

22. Lees AJ, Blackburn NA, Campbell VL. The nighttime problems of Parkinson's disease. *Clin Neuropharmacol*. 1988;11:512–519.

23. Olanow CW, Watts RL, Koller WC. An algorithm (decision tree) for the management of Parkinson's disease (2001): treatment guidelines. *Neurology*. 2001;56:S1–S88.

24. Chaudhuri KR, Healy DG, Schapira AHV. Non-motor symptoms of Parkinson's disease: diagnosis and management. *Lancet Neurol*. 2006;5:235–245.

25. Moro deCasillas ML, Riley D. Insomnia. In: Pfeiffer RF, Bodis-Wollner I, eds. *Parkinson's Disease and Nonmotor Dysfunction*. New York: Humana Press; 2005:181–189.

26. Ondo WG, Vuong KD, Jankovic J. Exploring the relationship between Parkinson disease and restless legs syndrome. *Arch Neurol*. 2002;59:421–424.

27. Paus S, Brecht HM, Koster J, Seeger G, Klockgether T, Wullner U. Sleep attacks, daytime sleepiness, and dopamine agonists in Parkinson's disease. *Mov Disord*. 2003;18:659–667.

28. Abbott RD, Petrovich H, White LR, et al. Frequency of bowel movements and the future risk of Parkinson's disease. *Neurology*. 2001;57:456–462.

Chapter 2

Diagnosis of Parkinson's disease

Indu Subramanian

Parkinsonism is a syndrome that presents with motor symptoms including tremor, bradykinesia (slowness of movement), rigidity, and postural instability. In general, to make a clinical diagnosis of parkinsonism the presence of at least two of four major signs is required: tremor at rest, rigidity, bradykinesia, and postural instability.

The clinical examination of the parkinsonian patient includes the following tests: Bradykinesia is tested by determining the speed and amplitude of motor tasks, such as how quickly the person can tap a finger and thumb together, or tap the foot up and down. Tremor is determined by inspection. The physician assesses rigidity by passively moving the neck, arms, and legs, feeling for resistance to movement, while the patient relaxes. Postural instability is tested with the "pull test" in which the examiner stands behind the patient and asks the patient to maintain balance when pulled backwards. The examiner pulls back briskly to assess the patient's ability to recover, being careful to prevent the patient from falling.

There are a number of causes of parkinsonism that stem from disruption of the dopaminergic nigrostriatal pathways. These causes include strokes, tumors, metabolic insults, and drugs. These are discussed in Chapter 3.

In contrast, idiopathic Parkinson's disease (PD) is a distinct disorder that has characteristic pathological findings of depigmentation in the neurons of the substantia nigra and deposition of Lewy bodies. Parkinson's disease is the most common form of parkinsonism, accounting for the majority of cases. The diagnosis of PD is based on clinical findings and does not rely on the use of specific diagnostic tests or biomarkers.

Diagnostic Criteria

Parkinson's disease must be clinically diagnosed due to the lack of neuroimaging or biomarkers for the disease. The definitive diagnosis of PD can only be made pathologically, but there are certain clinical criteria that have been proposed for the diagnosis of PD. The most widely used clinical criteria are the UK Brain Bank criteria (Table 2.1). These clinical criteria include the presence of bradykinesia and an additional sign of either rigidity, rest

Table 2.1 UK Parkinson's Disease Society Brain Bank clinical diagnostic criteria

Inclusion criteria

Bradykinesia and at least one of the following:

- Muscular rigidity
- 4 to 6 Hz rest tremor
- Postural instability not caused by primary visual, vestibular, cerebellar, or proprioceptive dysfunction

Exclusion criteria

History of repeated strokes with stepwise progression of Parkinson's features

History of repeated head injury

History of definite encephalitis

Oculogyric crises

Neuroleptic treatment at onset of symptoms

More than one affected relative

Sustained remission

Strictly unilateral features after 3 years

Supranuclear gaze palsy

Cerebellar signs

Early severe autonomic involvement

Early severe dementia with disturbances of memory, language, and praxis

Babinski's sign

Presence of cerebral tumor or communicating hydrocephalus on CT scan

Negative response to large doses of levodopa (if malabsorption is excluded)

MPTP exposure

Supportive criteria (three or more required for diagnosis of PD)

Unilateral onset

Rest tremor present

Progressive disorder

Persistent asymmetry affecting side of onset most

Excellent response (70% to 100%) to levodopa

Severe levodopa-induced chorea

Levodopa response for 5 years or more

Clinical course of 10 years or more

PD, Parkinson's disease. *Source*: Litvan I, Bhatia KP, Burn DJ, et al. Movement Disorders Society Scientific Issues Committee. Movement Disorders Society Scientific Issues Committee report: SIC Task Force appraisal of clinical diagnostic criteria for Parkinsonian disorders. *Mov Disord.* 2003;18(5):467–486. Reprinted with permission.

tremor, or postural instability. The next step includes exclusion of atypical features of parkinsonism, such as repeated strokes, repeated head injuries, strictly unilateral features after 3 years, early severe dementia, and so on. Finally, the presence of three or more supportive criteria such as unilateral onset of symptoms, presence of rest tremor, excellent response to levodopa, or severe levodopa-induced chorea, among others, should be used in confirming the diagnosis of PD.

Gelb et al.[1] devised another system, which classified patients into possible, probable, and definite PD. Patients with probable PD have clinical features that are absolutely typical of PD, at least 3 years of parkinsonian symptoms without development of atypical features, and a clear clinical response to dopaminergic therapy. Possible PD criteria are less strict and do not require as many typical features; symptom duration can be less than 3 years, and patients need not have received an adequate trial of dopaminergic therapy. Patients who do not respond to an adequate trial of dopaminergic therapy do not qualify for either possible or probable PD. Patients who have autopsy findings consistent with PD as defined by a specific set of histopathologic criteria and who meet all the criteria for possible PD are classified as definite PD.

Calne et al.[2] defined a purely clinically based classification system with three categories: clinically possible idiopathic parkinsonism (IP), clinically probable IP, and clinically definite IP. Clinically possible IP requires the presence of any one of the following: tremor, rigidity, or bradykinesia. The tremor must be of recent onset and may be postural or resting. Clinically probable IP requires a combination of any two of the following features: resting tremor, rigidity, bradykinesia, or impaired postural reflexes. Alternatively, asymmetrical resting tremor, asymmetrical rigidity, or asymmetrical bradykinesia are sufficient. Clinically definite IP requires any combination of three of the following features: resting tremor, rigidity, bradykinesia, or impaired postural reflexes. Alternatively sufficient are two of these features with one of the first three displaying asymmetry.

Helpful clinical features in making a diagnosis of PD include a rest tremor of the fingers, legs, or jaw associated with stiffness and slowness that affects one side of the body. However, even with such a classical picture, alternative diagnoses such as vascular or drug-induced parkinsonism may still be the culprit. A percentage of patients with PD do not have tremor at any stage in their disease, and other patients with PD may have tremor that resembles essential tremor for many years preceding the diagnosis of PD. Patients presenting with early falls or major balance problems within the first year of presentation are unlikely to have PD. Recurrent falling within the first year was a strong predictor of PSP, whereas time to onset of falling was more delayed in corticobasal degeneration (CBD), dementia with Lewy bodies (DLB), and multiple system atrophy (MSA), and was most prolonged in PD.[3] In another study differentiating PD from PSP and MSA, lack of tremor, symmetry, and rapid progression were more likely in the PSP and MSA groups. Patients with PD universally had a good levodopa response and lacked orthostatic hypotension.[4]

Diagnostic testing

Dopamine responsiveness has been proposed as a major supporting feature for the diagnosis of PD. The use of acute levodopa challenges in the office setting has been proposed to differentiate PD from atypical parkinsonian disorders. Others have proposed the use of apomorphine (a short-acting injectable dopamine agonist) to support the diagnosis of PD. A study was performed on 82 patients with undifferentiated parkinsonism who were pre-treated with domperidone to prevent peripheral dopaminergic side effects.[5] These patients were given an acute levodopa challenge of 250/25 mg of levodopa/carbidopa orally. A blinded rater assessed the Unified Parkinson's Disease Rating Scale scores at 15-minute intervals. An improvement of greater than 30% supported a diagnosis of PD. These patients were followed for 24 months and retested clinically. The UK Brain Bank criteria were used to diagnose PD. The acute levodopa challenge test had 71% sensitivity and 81% specificity for detecting patients with PD.[5] Another study showed a sensitivity of 77% and specificity of 71% for distinguishing PD from other forms of parkinsonism using apomorphine and levodopa challenges. The negative predictive value of such tests in a de novo patient is only between 40% and 60%. On the other hand, up to 20% of patients with atypical parkinsonism from MSA and vascular PD patients can respond to such challenges. Hence, the diagnostic accuracy of such testing in the office setting remains questionable. Patients who do not respond in the office setting should still undergo a trial of high doses (up to 1000 mg per day) of levodopa for a month or two if clinical suspicion of PD is high. Other diagnostic criteria such as stimulation of growth hormone with clonidine, olfaction testing, electro-oculography, and autonomic testing have been proposed. Diagnostic neuroimaging studies such as magnetic resonance imaging (MRI), sonography, single-photon emission computed tomography (SPECT), and positron emission tomography (PET) scans have also been reviewed.

An evidence-based review by the American Academy of Neurology Practice recommended that the following clinical features be considered in distinguishing PD from other parkinsonian syndromes: (1) falls at presentation and early in the disease course, (2) poor response to levodopa, (3) symmetry at onset, (4) rapid progression (to Hoehn and Yahr stage 3 in 3 years), (5) lack of tremor, and (6) dysautonomia (urinary urgency/incontinence, fecal incontinence, urinary retention requiring catheterization, persistent erectile failure, or symptomatic orthostatic hypotension). Levodopa challenges should be considered for confirmation when the diagnosis is in doubt. Olfaction testing should be considered to differentiate PD from PSP and CBD but not PD from MSA. Growth hormone stimulation, electro-oculography, and SPECT scans many not be useful, and there is insufficient evidence regarding urodynamics, autonomic testing, urethral and anal electromyogram, MRI, sonography, and PET scanning in differentiating PD from other forms of parkinsonism.[6]

Clinicopathologic studies

Parkinson's disease is commonly defined as progressive parkinsonism of unknown cause without features suggesting another diagnosis that responds to dopaminergic medications.

In making this clinical diagnosis, even when patients have been treated by movement disorder neurologists, the diagnosis was incorrect in up to

24% of cases when evaluated in a clinicopathologic series. In a prospective clinicopathologic series, Rajput et al.[7] showed that initial clinical diagnosis within 5 years of disease onset was correct in only 65% of cases, and after a mean follow-up of 12 years, the final diagnosis of PD was confirmed at autopsy in 76% of cases. PD was diagnosed if patients had at least two of the three nonpostural signs (bradykinesia, rigidity, and rest tremor), no identifiable cause of parkinsonism, and no clinical evidence of wide-spread central nervous system lesions. Early untreated PD patients who were enrolled in the **D**eprenyl **a**nd **T**ocopherol **A**ntioxidative **T**herapy **of P**arkinsonism (DATATOP) study were reevaluated to assess the evolution of their diagnosis over time. Approximately 8% to 9% of cases were thought to have another cause for the parkinsonism. Clinical features that led to diagnoses other than PD included higher Hoehn and Yahr stage, higher Unified Parkinson's Disease Rating Scale (UPDRS) scores for bradykinesia, postural instability and gait difficulty, and a lower tremor score (Table 2.2).[8]

The UK Brain Bank has been collecting brain tissue from patients with PD for decades and has amassed a large prospective clinical and pathological follow-up on PD patients. Even with such criteria, up to 10% of patients diagnosed with PD were reassigned to another diagnosis on autopsy. Initial reports from 1991 showed a diagnostic accuracy of 76%. This group utilized the UK Brain Bank criteria on 100 more patients with clinicopathologic correlations and published their data in 2001.[9] They reported a diagnostic accuracy rate of 90% and credited this improved rate to a greater aware-ness among clinicians of the pitfalls of diagnosing PD and distinguishing PD from other disorders. Other diagnoses often included so-called parkinson-plus disorders such as PSP, CBD, MSA or essential tremor, and vascular parkinsonism or drug-induced parkinsonism. There is additional contr-oversy over the existence of DLB as a separate disease entity.[10]

Rating scales

Standardized rating scales have been implemented for quantifying dis-ease severity, motor symptoms, and quality of life. As these scales can change depending on whether the patient is "on" or "off" medications for Parkinson's disease, an additional qualifier is the state in which the patient is seen. Videotaping patients, having them fill out motor symptom diaries, and timed testing of maneuvers such as timed walking tests are also used, especially in clinical trials. All of the following scales have been validated and appear to have good inter-rater and intra-rater reliability.

Hoehn and Yahr scale
This scale was described over 30 years ago, in the pre-levodopa era, but is still used widely. In the early 1990s 0.5 increments were added for use in some clinical trials. This scale provides an overall assessment of severity based on clinical features and functional disability. The main focus of the scale is dif-ferentiating unilateral versus bilateral symptoms and presence or absence of

balance issues. It has many shortcomings but remains a useful scale, especially in determining inclusion/exclusion criteria for clinical trials.[11]

Schwab and England's Activities of Daily Living scale (Table 2.2) is a 10-point scale that looks at the level of disability in performing activities of daily living. A score of 100% stands for normal function and 0% represents total dependency.

Unified Parkinson's disease rating scale

This scale has been recently modified into the "new" UPDRS, which is being validated against the conventional UPDRS.[12] Studies to date have used the original version. There are four components to this scale: Part I,

Table 2.2 Unified Parkinson's disease rating scale
I. Mentation, behavior, and mood
1. Intellectual impairment
0 = None
1 = Mild; consistent forgetfulness with partial recollection of events and no other difficulties
2 = Moderate memory loss, with disorientation and moderate difficulty handling complex problems; mild but definite impairment of function at home with need of occasional prompting
3 = Severe memory loss with disorientation for time and often to place; severe impairment in handling problems
4 = Severe memory loss with orientation preserved to person only; unable to make judgments or solve problems; requires much help with personal care; cannot be left alone at all
2. Thought disorder (due to dementia or drug intoxication)
0 = None
1 = Vivid dreaming
2 = "Benign" hallucinations with insight retained
3 = Occasional to frequent hallucinations or delusions; without insight; could interfere with daily activities
4 = Persistent hallucinations, delusions, or florid psychosis; not able to care for self
3. Depression
0 = None
1 = Periods of sadness or guilt greater than normal, never sustained for days or weeks
2 = Sustained depression (1 week or more)
3 = Sustained depression with vegetative symptoms (insomnia, anorexia, weight loss, loss of interest)
4 = Sustained depression with vegetative symptoms and suicidal thoughts or intent
4. Motivation/initiative
0 = Normal
1 = Less assertive than usual; more passive
2 = Loss of initiative or disinterest in elective (nonroutine) activities
3 = Loss of initiative or disinterest in day-to-day (routine) activities
4 = Withdrawn, complete loss of motivation

Table 2.2 *continued*

II. Activities of daily living (for both "on" and "off")

5. Speech
   - 0 = Normal
   - 1 = Mildly affected; no difficulty being understood
   - 2 = Moderately affected; sometimes asked to repeat statements
   - 3 = Severely affected; frequently asked to repeat statements
   - 4 = Unintelligible most of the time

6. Salivation
   - 0 = Normal
   - 1 = Slight but definite excess of saliva in mouth; may have nighttime drooling
   - 2 = Moderately excessive saliva; may have minimal drooling
   - 3 = Marked excess of saliva with some drooling
   - 4 = Marked drooling, requires constant tissue or handkerchief

7. Swallowing
   - 0 = Normal
   - 1 = Rare choking
   - 2 = Occasional choking
   - 3 = Requires soft food
   - 4 = Requires NG tube or gastrostomy feeding

8. Handwriting
   - 0 = Normal
   - 1 = Slightly slow or small
   - 2 = Moderately slow or small; all words are legible
   - 3 = Severely affected; not all words are legible
   - 4 = The majority of words are not legible

9. Cutting food and handling utensils
   - 0 = Normal
   - 1 = Somewhat slow and clumsy, but no help needed
   - 2 = Can cut most foods, although clumsy and slow; some help needed
   - 3 = Food must be cut by someone, but can still feed slowly
   - 4 = Needs to be fed

10. Dressing
    - 0 = Normal
    - 1 = Somewhat slow, but no help needed
    - 2 = Occasional assistance with buttoning, getting arms in sleeves
    - 3 = Considerable help required, but can do some things alone
    - 4 = Helpless

11. Hygiene
    - 0 = Normal
    - 1 = Somewhat slow, but no help needed
    - 2 = Needs help to shower or bathe, or very slow in hygienic care
    - 3 = Requires assistance for washing, brushing teeth, combing hair, going to bathroom
    - 4 = Foley catheter or other mechanical aids

Table 2.2 *continued*

12. Turning in bed and adjusting bed clothes

    0 = Normal

    1 = Somewhat slow and clumsy, but no help needed

    2 = Can turn alone or adjust sheets, but with great difficulty

    3 = Can initiate, but not turn or adjust sheets alone

    4 = Helpless

13. Falling (unrelated to freezing)

    0 = None

    1 = Rare falling

    2 = Occasionally falls, less than once per day

    3 = Falls an average of once daily

    4 = Falls more than once daily

14. Freezing when walking

    0 = None

    1 = Rare freezing when walking; may have start hesitation

    2 = Occasional freezing when walking

    3 = Frequent freezing; occasional falls from freezing

    4 = Frequent falls from freezing

15. Walking

    0 = Normal

    1 = Mild difficulty; may not swing arms or may tend to drag leg

    2 = Moderate difficulty, but requires little or no assistance

    3 = Severe disturbance of walking requiring assistance

    4 = Cannot walk at all, even with assistance

16. Tremor (symptomatic complaint of tremor in any part of body)

    0 = Absent

    1 = Slight and infrequently present

    2 = Moderate; bothersome to patient

    3 = Severe; interferes with many activities

    4 = Marked; interferes with most activities

17. Sensory complaints related to parkinsonism

    0 = None

    1 = Occasionally has numbness, tingling, or mild aching

    2 = Frequently has numbness, tingling, or aching; not distressing

    3 = Frequent painful sensations

    4 = Excruciating pain

III. Motor examination

18. Speech

    0 = Normal

    1 = Slight loss of expression, diction, and/or volume

    2 = Monotone, slurred but understandable; moderately impaired

    3 = Marked impairment, difficult to understand

    4 = Unintelligible

Table 2.2 *continued*

19. Facial expression

    0 = Normal

    1 = Minimal hypomimia, could be normal "poker face"

    2 = Slight but definitely abnormal diminution of facial expression

    3 = Moderate hypomimia; lips parted some of the time

    4 = Masked or fixed facies with severe or complete loss of facial expression; lips parted one-quarter inch or more

20. Tremor at rest (head, upper and lower extremities)

    0 = Absent

    1 = Slight and infrequently present

    2 = Mild in amplitude and persistent, or moderate in amplitude but only intermittently present

    3 = Moderate in amplitude and present most of the time

    4 = Marked in amplitude and present most of the time

21. Action or postural tremor of hands

    0 = Absent

    1 = Slight; present with action

    2 = Moderate in amplitude, present with action

    3 = Moderate in amplitude with posture holding as well as action

    4 = Marked in amplitude; interferes with feeding

22. Rigidity (judged on passive movement of major joints with patient relaxed in sitting position; cogwheeling to be ignored)

    0 = Absent

    1 = Slight or detectable only when activated by mirror or other movements

    2 = Mild to moderate

    3 = Marked, but full range of motion easily achieved

    4 = Severe, range of motion achieved with difficulty

23. Finger taps (patient taps thumb with index finger in rapid succession)

    0 = Normal

    1 = Mild slowing and/or reduction in amplitude

    2 = Moderately impaired; definite and early fatiguing; may have occasional arrests in movement

    3 = Severely impaired; frequent hesitation in initiating movements or arrests in ongoing movement

    4 = Can barely perform the task

24. Hand movements (patient opens and closes hands in rapid succession)

    0 = Normal

    1 = Mild slowing and/or reduction in amplitude

    2 = Moderately impaired; definite and early fatiguing; may have occasional arrests in movement

    3 = Severely impaired; frequent hesitation in initiating movements or arrests in ongoing movement

    4 = Can barely perform the task

Table 2.2 *continued*

25. Rapid alternating movements of hands (pronation-supination movements of hands, vertically and horizontally, with as large an amplitude as possible, both hands simultaneously)

   0 = Normal

   1 = Mild slowing and/or reduction in amplitude

   2 = Moderately impaired; definite and early fatiguing; may have occasional arrests in movement

   3 = Severely impaired; frequent hesitation in initiating movements or arrests in ongoing movement

   4 = Can barely perform the task

26. Leg agility (patient taps heel on the ground in rapid succession, picking up entire leg; amplitude should be at least 3 inches)

   0 = Normal

   1 = Mild slowing and/or reduction in amplitude

   2 = Moderately impaired; definite and early fatiguing; may have occasional arrests in movement

   3 = Severely impaired; frequent hesitation in initiating movements or arrests in ongoing movement

   4 = Can barely perform the task

27. Arising from chair (patient attempts to rise from a straight-backed chair, with arms folded across chest)

   0 = Normal

   1 = Slow, or may need more than one attempt

   2 = Pushes self up from arms of seat

   3 = Tends to fall back and may have to try more than one time, but can get up without help

   4 = Unable to rise without help

28. Posture

   0 = Normal, erect

   1 = Not quite erect, slightly stooped posture; could be normal for older person

   2 = Moderately stooped posture, definitely abnormal; may be slightly leaning to one side

   3 = Severely stooped posture with kyphosis; may be moderately leaning to one side

   4 = Marked flexion with extreme abnormality of posture

29. Gait

   0 = Normal

   1 = Walks slowly, may shuffle with short steps, but no festination (hastening steps) or propulsion

   2 = Walks with difficulty, but requires little or no assistance; may have some festination, short steps, or propulsion

   3 = Severe disturbance of gait requiring assistance

   4 = Cannot walk at all, even with assistance

30. Postural stability (response to sudden, strong posterior displacement produced by pull on shoulders while patient is erect with eyes open and feet slightly apart; patient is prepared)

   0 = Normal

   1 = Retropulsion, but recovers unaided

Table 2.2 *continued*

2 = Absence of postural response; would fall if not caught by examiner

3 = Very unstable, tends to lose balance spontaneously

4 = Unable to stand without assistance

31. Body bradykinesia and hypokinesia (combining slowness, hesitancy, decreased arm swing, small amplitude, and poverty of movement in general)

   0 = None

   1 = Minimal slowness, giving movement a deliberate character; could be normal for some persons; possibly reduced amplitude

   2 = Mild degree of slowness and poverty of movement that is definitely abnormal; alternatively, some reduced amplitude

   3 = Moderate slowness, poverty or small amplitude of movement

   4 = Marked slowness, poverty or small amplitude of movement

IV. Complications of therapy (in the past week)

Dyskinesias

32. Duration: What proportion of the waking day are dyskinesias present? (historical information)

   0 = None

   1 = 1% to 25% of day

   2 = 26% to 50% of day

   3 = 51% to 75% of day

   4 = 76% to 100% of day

33. Disability: How disabling are the dyskinesias? (historical information; may be modified by office examination)

   0 = Not disabling

   1 = Mildly disabling

   2 = Moderately disabling

   3 = Severely disabling

   4 = Completely disabling

34. Painful dyskinesias: How painful are the dyskinesias?

   0 = No painful dyskinesias

   1 = Slight

   2 = Moderate

   3 = Severe

   4 = Marked

35. Presence of early morning dystonia (historical information)

   0 = No

   1 = Yes

Clinical fluctuations

36. Are "off" periods predictable?

   0 = No

   1 = Yes

37. Are "off" periods unpredictable?

   0 = No

   1 = Yes

Table 2.2 *continued*

38. Do "off" periods come on suddenly, within a few seconds?

    0 = No

    1 = Yes

39. What proportion of the waking day is the patient "off" on average?

    0 = None

    1 = 1% to 25% of day

    2 = 26% to 50% of day

    3 = 51% to 75% of day

    4 = 76% to 100% of day

Other complications

40. Does the patient have anorexia, nausea, or vomiting?

    0 = No

    1 = Yes

41. Any sleep disturbances, such as insomnia or hypersomnolence?

    0 = No

    1 = Yes

42. Does the patient have symptomatic orthostasis? (Record the patient's blood pressure, height, and weight on the scoring form)

    0 = No

    1 = Yes

V. Modified Hoehn and Yahr staging

Stage 0 = No signs of disease

Stage 1 = Unilateral disease

Stage 1.5 = Unilateral plus axial involvement

Stage 2 = Bilateral disease, without impairment of balance

Stage 2.5 = Mild bilateral disease, with recovery on pull test

Stage 3 = Mild to moderate bilateral disease; some postural instability; physically independent

Stage 4 = Severe disability; still able to walk or stand unassisted

Stage 5 = Wheelchair bound or bedridden unless aided

VI. Schwab and England Activities of Daily Living scale

100% = Completely independent: able to do all chores without slowness, difficulty, or impairment; essentially normal; unaware of any difficulty

90% = Completely independent: able to do all chores with some degree of slowness, difficulty, and impairment; might take twice as long; beginning to be aware of difficulty

80% = Completely independent in most chores: takes twice as long; conscious of difficulty and slowness

70% = Not completely independent: more difficulty with some chores, 3 to 4 times as long in some; must spend a large part of the day with chores

60% = Some dependency: can do most chores, but exceedingly slowly and with much effort; errors; some chores impossible

50% = More dependent: help with half, slower, etc.; difficulty with everything

40% = Very dependent: can assist with all chores, but can complete few alone

30% = With effort, now and then does a few chores alone or begins alone; much help needed

Table 2.2 *continued*
20% = Nothing alone; can be a slight help with some chores; severe invalid
10% = Totally dependent, helpless; complete invalid
0% = Vegetative functions such as swallowing, bladder and bowel functions are not functioning; bedridden

Source: Fahn S, Elton RL. Unified Parkinson's disease rating scale. In: Fahn S, Marsden CD, Goldstein M, Calne DB, eds. *Recent Developments in Parkinson's Disease*, Vol. 2. Florham Park, NJ: Macmillan Healthcare Information; 1987:153–163, 293–304. Reprinted with permission.

mentation, behavior, and mood; Part II, activities of daily living; Part III, motor examination; and Part IV, complications.

Part I deals with issues such as dementia, depression, apathy, and psychosis. Part II focuses on the patient's ability to perform activities in his or her daily life such as dressing, grooming, turning in bed, and using utensils. Part III is rated by the examiner and measures the cardinal motor features such as speech, facial expression, tremor, tone, slowness of movement in the hands and legs, walking, and balance. Part IV measures the complications of treatment including questions on dyskinesias and dystonia. The Hoehn and Yahr and Schwab and England scales are also included in the full version of the UPDRS as Parts V and VI, respectively. An educational videotape and a standardized test have been developed that allow for improved inter-rater reliability. A concern that certain nonmotor aspects of Parkinson's disease were not captured in the older version led to the addition of these features in the updated UPDRS. Questions to better rate dyskinesias were also incorporated.[13]

Summary

PD is a clinical diagnosis based on the cardinal features of bradykinesia, rigidity, rest tremor, and postural instability. The UK Brain Bank criteria are the most commonly used clinical diagnostic criteria for this diagnosis. Clinicopathologic studies have shown that a premortem diagnosis of PD can be made in greater than 90% of cases. Although there are a number of rating scales available to assess the severity of PD, these are mainly used in clinical trials.

References

1. Gelb DJ, Oliver E, Gilman S. Diagnostic criteria for Parkinson disease. *Arch Neurol.* 1999;56(1):33–39.

2. Calne DB, Snow BJ, Lee C. Criteria for diagnosing Parkinson's disease. *Ann Neurol.* 1992;32(suppl):S125–S127.

3. Wenning GK, Ebersbach G, Verny M, et al. Progression of falls in postmortem-confirmed parkinsonian disorders. *Mov Disord.* 1999;14(6):947–950.

4. Colosimo C, Albanese A, Hughes AJ, de Bruin VM, Lees AJ. Some specific clinical features differentiate multiple system atrophy (striatonigral variety) from Parkinson's disease. *Arch Neurol.* 1995;52(3):294–298.

5. Merello M, Nouzeilles MI, Arce GP, Leiguarda R. Accuracy of acute levodopa challenge for clinical prediction of sustained long-term levodopa response as a major criterion for idiopathic Parkinson's disease diagnosis. *Mov Disord.* 2002;17(4):795–798.

6. Suchowersky O, Reich S, Perlmutter J, Zesiewicz T, Gronseth G, Weiner WJ. Practice parameter: diagnosis and prognosis of new onset Parkinson disease (an evidence-based review). Report of the Quality Standards Subcommittee of the American Academy of Neurology. *Neurology.* 2006;66(7):968–975.

7. Rajput AH, Rozdilsky B, Rajput A. Accuracy of clinical diagnosis in parkinsonism—a prospective study. *Can J Neurol Sci.* 1991;18(3):275–278.

8. Jankovic J, Rajput AH, McDermott MP, Perl DP. The evolution of diagnosis in early Parkinson disease. Parkinson Study Group. *Arch Neurol.* 2000;57(3):369–72.

9. Hughes AJ, Ben-Shlomo Y, Daniel SE, Lees AJ. What features improve the accuracy of clinical diagnosis in Parkinson's disease: a clinicopathologic study. *Neurology.* 2001;57(10 suppl 3):S34–S38.

10. Litvan I, Bhatia KP, Burn DJ, et al. Movement Disorders Society Scientific Issues Committee report: SIC task force appraisal of clinical diagnostic criteria for Parkinsonian disorders. *Mov Disord.* 2003;18(5):467–486.

11. Fahn S, Elton RL. Unified parkinson's disease rating scale. In: Fahn S, Marsden CD, Goldstein M, Calne DB, eds. *Recent Developments in Parkinson's Disease.* Vol. 2. Florham Park, NJ: Macmillan Healthcare Information; 1987:153–163, 293–304.

12. Goetz CG, Poewe W, Rascol O, et al. Movement Disorder Society Task Force report on the Hoehn and Yahr staging scale: status and recommendations. *Mov Disord.* 2004;19(9):1020–1028.

13. Goetz CG, Fahn S, Martinez-Martin P, et al. Movement Disorder Society sponsored revision of the Unified Parkinson's Disease Rating Scale (MDS-UPDRS): process, format, and clinimetric testing plan. *Mov Disord.* 2007;22(1):41–47.

Chapter 3

Differential diagnosis

Ariane Park and Cindy Zadikoff

Parkinsonism is characterized by tremor, akinesia (or bradykinesia), rigidity, and postural instability. While idiopathic Parkinson's disease (PD) is the most common cause of parkinsonism, there are a wide range of other diseases that can also cause parkinsonism. In fact, approximately 25% of patients initially diagnosed with PD are found to have parkinsonism as part of another disorder.[12] As therapeutic advances are made, it becomes increasingly important to not only recognize PD in its early stages but also distinguish PD from other causes of parkinsonism. Therefore, it is important to recognize some of the unique features that can help distinguish between the different causes of parkinsonism.

Broadly, causes of parkinsonism can be grouped into primary (or idiopathic), secondary (or symptomatic), and neurodegenerative diseases, including parkinsonism-plus syndromes (Table 3.1). This chapter reviews some of the more common atypical features ("red flags") that should raise suspicion that one is not dealing with idiopathic PD, and discusses the major entities that should be considered in the differential diagnosis of idiopathic PD.

Table 3.1 Classification of parkinsonism

Primary (idiopathic)

Parkinson's disease

Juvenile parkinsonism

Secondary (acquired, symptomatic)

Infectious: postencephalitic, syphilis, HIV, Creutzfeldt-Jakob disease

Drugs: dopamine-receptor blocking drugs (antipsychotic, antiemetic drugs), reserpine, tetrabenazine, alpha-methyl-dopa, lithium, flunarizine, cinnarizine

Toxins: MPTP, carbon monoxide, cobalt, cyanide, manganese, methanol, ethanol

Vascular: multi-infarct

Trauma: pugilistic encephalopathy

Metabolic: hypoparathyroidism with basal ganglia calcification, hypothyroidism, hepatocerebral degeneration, Wilson's disease, neurodegeneration with brain iron accumulation (formerly Hallervorden-Spatz disease), dopa-responsive dystonia

Mitochondrial cytopathies

Other: brain tumor, normal pressure hydrocephalus, syringomesencephatia

Table 3.1 *continued*
Neurodegenerative
Progressive supranuclear palsy
Multiple system atrophy
Corticobasal ganglionic degeneration
Dementia with Lewy bodies
Huntington's disease
Frontotemporal dementia and parkinsonism linked to chromosome 17
Spinocerebellar ataxias (especially Machado-Joseph disease)
Neuroacanthocytosis
Parkinsonism-dementia-amyotrophic lateral sclerosis complex of Guam
X-linked dystonia-Parkinsonism (Lubag)
Alzheimer's disease

Atypical features ("red flags")

Not all cases of PD demonstrate the classic signs, and any atypical features should suggest the possibility of a different parkinsonian syndrome. A thorough history and physical examination remain the most important factors in establishing a correct diagnosis. The history should include not only the precise chronology of symptoms but also information regarding medications and responses to therapies, as well as family history of neurological diseases. The examination should include a search for the classical features of PD as well as for any signs that might point to a different etiology.

Postural instability

Postural instability and falls are not prominent early in the course of PD and, when found, should point to another cause of parkinsonism. If a patient presents with these signs soon after disease onset, the clinician should consider an alternative diagnosis such as progressive supranuclear palsy (PSP) or multiple system atrophy (MSA). The incidence of recurrent falls within the first year has been shown to be a strong predictor of PSP (68% of pathologically confirmed cases).[3] Normal pressure hydrocephalus should also be included in the differential if the postural instability is associated with urinary incontinence and dementia.

Dementia

While PD patients can develop dementia, they do not typically present with early dementia. Therefore, in patients with early dementia and parkinsonian features, dementia with Lewy bodies (DLB) should be considered. Other atypical syndromes that can present with early cognitive problems include PSP, corticobasal degeneration (CBD), and frontotemporal dementia with parkinsonism.

Tremor

The classic tremor of PD begins as an asymmetric resting tremor (often of the hand), which attenuates with voluntary movement and often emerges when walking. The presence of an asymmetric resting tremor is quite specific for idiopathic PD, although it can occur occasionally in MSA or even PSP. While its absence does not rule out idiopathic PD, lack of an asymmetrical resting tremor in the company of other atypical features should suggest a different cause of parkinsonism.

A postural and action tremor, on the other hand, is a common, nonspecific feature seen in many of the parkinsonian disorders. A tremor with a jerky quality can be seen in both MSA and CBD and often is indicative of the coexistence of myoclonus. It is also important to mention that although essential tremor (ET) is sometimes confused with early PD, these two tremors are typically easy to distinguish from each other clinically. ET is characterized by a symmetrical postural/action tremor that is often accompanied by head and voice tremors, and the handwriting in ET patients is often large and tremulous. PD patients, on the other hand, may have a jaw or chin tremor; however, they rarely display a head or vocal tremor, and their handwriting is classically micrographic. Furthermore, rigidity and bradykinesia are not associated with ET.

Symmetry

PD signs are usually unilateral early in the disease course, but then become bilateral within several years. In the other atypical parkinsonian disorders, the onset is usually bilateral. However, in patients with markedly asymmetrical motor signs, one must consider CBD or hemiparkinsonism-hemiatrophy (HPHA). HPHA is a rare disorder seen in younger populations in whom there may be a history of perinatal hypoxic-ischemic injury.[4] HPHA is associated with unilateral body atrophy (face, arm, or leg), ipsilateral parkinsonism with early-onset dystonia, slow progression, and poor response to levodopa.

Dysautonomia

Early and severe autonomic dysfunction is atypical for PD. However, it tends to be prominent in MSA and is an important diagnostic feature for it. Autonomic dysfunction in MSA typically consists of orthostatic hypotension, urinary dysfunction, and, in almost all men, erectile dysfunction or impotence. Another study showed that symptomatic orthostatic hypotension occurring within the first year of disease predicted MSA in 75% of pathologically confirmed cases.[5] However, none of these dysautonomic features are specific for MSA, as patients with PD, PSP, and DLB can demonstrate similar findings during the course of disease.

Eye movement abnormalities

Eye movement abnormalities are generally absent in PD. If eye movement dysfunction is noted on exam, one should consider other disorders. One of the cardinal manifestations of PSP is supranuclear ophthalmoplegia (SNO), which usually starts with slowing of vertical saccades and eventually leads to a supranuclear gaze palsy—specifically, downward gaze restriction.

While downward gaze restriction is not seen in PD, upward gaze limitation can be seen in both PSP and PD, and can also be seen with normal aging. A supranuclear gaze palsy can also been seen in CBD; however, while saccade velocity is usually preserved, saccade latency is increased as compared to PSP.[6] Other diseases in which supranuclear gaze palsy may also be seen include DLB, vascular parkinsonism, Creutzfeld-Jakob disease, and Huntington's disease.

Other cortical signs

Cortical signs are not a hallmark of PD. In fact, evidence of cortical involvement such as aphasia and apraxia are part of the exclusion criteria based on the UK Brain Bank criteria.[1] If apraxia, cortical sensory loss, alien limb phenomenon, or corticospinal tract findings are seen, one must consider one of the parkinsonism-plus syndromes, particularly CBD. In CBD these signs tend to be asymmetrical initially but then eventually progress to both sides. Language disorders can be seen in CBD, frontotemporal dementias, and Alzheimer's disease.

Response to levodopa

PD patients have a sustained good symptomatic benefit from levodopa, despite the eventual development of motor complications, including wearing-off and dyskinesias. In fact, excellent response to levodopa for 5 years or more and levodopa-induced dyskinesias are among the supportive criteria for the diagnosis of definite PD.[3] In one study, when patients with parkinsonian symptoms were given an acute levodopa challenge, the sensitivity for predicting the eventual diagnosis of PD was 70.9%, and the specificity was 81.4%.[7] A poor or absent response to high doses of levodopa (up to 1000 mg per day) should be a red flag that another cause of parkinsonism is at hand. Patients with MSA may have a good initial response to levodopa, but this is not typically sustained. PSP and CBD patients do not respond to levodopa. Patients with DLB have a variable response to levodopa.

Other atypical features that should raise suspicion of other causes of parkinsonism include ataxia, pyramidal signs, neuropathy, and myoclonus.

Common diseases in the differential diagnosis of idiopathic PD

Tests are used as supportive evidence in diagnosing one of the atypical syndromes, but in many cases the findings are neither specific nor sensitive to them. The absence of findings on ancillary testing cannot rule out the diagnosis in question, and therefore these tests should only be used to support, and not make, a diagnosis.

Progressive supranuclear palsy

Epidemiology

PSP was first described by Steele, Richardson, and Olszewski in 1964. Recent epidemiological studies done in the UK have demonstrated a prevalence ranging from 3.1 to 6.4 per 100,000.[8,9] It is slightly more common in men with a mean age of onset of 62 years (range 55 to 70 years). Median survival from time of diagnosis is usually 6 to 9 years.[10]

Clinical characteristics

In advanced disease, PSP is relatively easy to diagnose; however, it can be challenging to diagnose in the early stages when some of the characteristic findings, such as supranuclear gaze palsy, have not emerged, or if other unusual signs predominate. The cardinal manifestations of PSP include parkinsonism, SNO, gait disturbances, and falls. SNO is the most distinguishing feature of PSP and is first manifested by slowing of vertical saccades, ultimately resulting in paralysis of voluntary downward gaze. The presence of SNO helps to establish the diagnosis of PSP; however, it is not always the first sign and may take months or even years to appear. In fact, Birdi et al.[10] reported that the gaze palsy did not appear during life in 50% of autopsy-confirmed cases. Other features include pseudo-bulbar palsy and behavioral and cognitive disturbances, including disinhibition and frontal lobe dysfunction. PSP patients often have an anxious, astonished look with deepened nasolabial folds and brow furrowing. Axial rigidity is more pronounced than appendicular rigidity and a less common, but classic, feature is extensor neck posturing. Finally, as opposed to the stooped posture seen in PD, PSP patients tend to be upright. In 1996, the National Institute of Neurological Disorders and Stroke and the Society for Progressive Supranuclear Palsy, Inc. (NINDS-SPSP), published diagnostic criteria for PSP (Table 3.2).[10] These criteria have high sensitivity, specificity, and positive predictive value. As with the majority of entities to be discussed here, a definite diagnosis of PSP relies on neuropathologic confirmation. However, a diagnosis of possible or probable PSP can be made based on these clinical criteria.

Ancillary tests

There is no diagnostic test for PSP. Neuroimaging features may be helpful; the main abnormality on brain MRI is midbrain atrophy. Other findings include increased signal in the midbrain, dilatation of the third ventricle, atrophy or increased signal of the red nucleus, and frontal or temporal atrophy. There is some evidence that the different parkinsonian syndromes have different brain-stem auditory startle responses, and this may be helpful diagnostically. One study demonstrated that patients with PSP had an absent or reduced auditory startle response of short latency and duration, low amplitude, and poor habituation. DLB patients had fewer responses with prolonged latency and normal habituation, and MSA patients had frequent, exaggerated responses of short latency, large amplitude, long duration, and lack of habituation.

Multiple system atrophy

Epidemiology

MSA is a sporadic neurodegenerative disease that is characterized by varying degrees of parkinsonism, cerebellar dysfunction, and autonomic insufficiency. There have been very few epidemiological studies reporting the incidence

Table 3.2 NINDS-SPSP clinical criteria for the diagnosis of PSP

Diagnostic categories	Inclusion criteria	Exclusion criteria	Supportive criteria
Possible and probable	Gradually progressive disorder with age at onset 40 or later	Recent history of encephalitis; alien limb syndrome; cortical sensory deficits; focal frontal or temporoparietal atrophy; hallucinations or delusions unrelated to dopaminergic therapy; cortical dementia of Alzheimer type; prominent, early cerebellar symptoms or unexplained dysautonomia; or evidence of other diseases that could explain the clinical features	Symmetric akinesia or rigidity, proximal more than distal; abnormal neck posture, especially retrocollis; poor or absent response of parkinsonism to levodopa; early dysphagia and dysarthria; early onset of cognitive impairment including more than two of the following: apathy, impairment in abstract thought, decreased verbal fluency, utilization or imitation behavior, or frontal release signs
Possible	Either vertical supranuclear palsy or both slowing of vertical saccades and postural instability with falls more than 1 year after disease onset		
Probable	Vertical supranuclear palsy and prominent postural instability with falls within first year of disease onset[a]		
Definite	All criteria for possible or probable PSP are met; histopathologic confirmation at autopsy		

[a] Later defined as falls or the tendency to fall (patients are able to stabilize themselves).

NINDS-SPSP, National Institute of Neurological Disorders and Stroke and Society for Progressive Supranuclear Palsy, Inc.; PSP, progressive supranuclear palsy. *Source*: Litvan I, Agid Y, Calne D, et al. Clinical research criteria for the diagnosis of progressive supranuclear palsy (Steele-Richardson-Olszewski syndrome): report of the NINDS-SPSP international workshop. *Neurology*. 1996;47:1–9. Reprinted with permission.

and prevalence of MSA. Schrag et al.[8] reported a prevalence of 4.4 per 100,000. The mean age of onset is 54.2 years with a survival of 6.2 years.[11]

Clinical characteristics

The terms *striatonigral degeneration*, *Shy-Drager syndrome*, and *olivoponto-cerebellar atrophy* previously referred to various forms of MSA. In 1998, a consensus committee developed diagnostic criteria for MSA based on four clinical domains: autonomic and urinary dysfunction, parkinsonism, cerebellar dysfunction, and corticospinal tract dysfunction (Table 3.3).[12] Based on this, the current nomenclature is MSA-P, where parkinsonism is more prominent and MSA-C, where cerebellar dysfunction is more prominent.

Common to both MSA-P and MSA-C is the presence of autonomic dysfunction. While patients with PD often have autonomic dysfunction, its presence early in the disease course, especially if severe, should raise the suspicion for MSA. It is important to note that many patients with MSA will initially have a good response to levodopa; however, they routinely lose this response over time, whereas patients with idiopathic PD maintain this response throughout the disease course. The appearance of cranial dystonia after the introduction of levodopa and anterocollis suggests a diagnosis of MSA rather than PD. Pyramidal signs such as brisk tendon reflexes may be present. Patients with MSA tend to become wheelchair bound quite

Table 3.3 Consensus criteria for the diagnosis of MSA

Clinical domain	Features	Criteria
Autonomic and urinary dysfunction	Orthostatic hypotension (by 20 mmHg systolic or 10 mmHg diastolic); urinary incontinence of incomplete bladder emptying	Orthostatic fall in blood pressure (by 30 mmHg systolic or 15 mmHg diastolic) and/or urinary incontinence (persistent, involuntary partial or total bladder emptying, accompanied by erectile dysfunction in men)[a]
Parkinsonism	Bradykinesias, rigidity, postural instability, and tremor	1 of 3 (rigidity, postural instability, and tremor) and bradykinesia
Cerebellar dysfunction	Gait ataxia; ataxic dysarthria; limb ataxia; sustained gaze-evoked nystagmus	Gait ataxia plus at least one other feature
Corticospinal tract dysfunction	Extensor plantar responses with hyperreflexia	No corticospinal tract features are used in defining the diagnosis of MSA[b]

[a] Note the different figures for orthostatic hypotension depending on whether it is used as a feature or a criterion.

[b] This criterion is ambiguously worded. One possible interpretation is that while corticospinal tract dysfunction can be used as a *feature* (characteristic of the disease), it cannot be used as a *criterion* (defining feature or composite of features required for diagnosis) in defining the diagnosis of MSA. The other interpretation is that corticospinal tract dysfunction cannot be used at all in consensus diagnostic criteria, in which case there may be no point mentioning it.

Source: Gilman S, Low PA, Quinn N, et al. Consensus statement on the diagnosis of multiple system atrophy. *J Neurol Sci.* 1999;163:94–98. Reprinted with permission.

rapidly. Finally, significant cognitive complaints in the setting of MSA are extremely rare and should point to a different parkinsonism-plus syndrome such as PSP or DLB.

Ancillary tests

The MRI of the brain findings in MSA-P include putaminal atrophy and abnormal putaminal hypointensity on T_2-weighted imaging with hyperintensity on the lateral edge. Histopathologic correlation studies suggest that these abnormalities represent neuronal loss, iron deposition, microgliosis, and astrocytosis in the putamen.[12] Another study found putaminal abnormalities on diffusion-weighted imaging, namely higher putaminal regional apparent diffusion coefficients, in MSA-P compared to PD.[13] The MRI findings for MSA-C include atrophy of the medulla, middle cerebellar peduncles, pons, and inferior olives and cerebellum. In addition, there may be increased signal in these regions. Other testing that can be useful for diagnosis include autonomic testing, anal sphincter electromyogram, and cardiac nuclear MIBG scans.[14]

Dementia with Lewy bodies

Epidemiology

Autopsy studies have shown that the prevalence of DLB in demented patients ranges from 15% to 25%,[15] making DLB the second most common cause of dementia, after Alzheimer's disease. The risk for developing dementia is up to six times higher in patients with idiopathic PD compared to the general population.[16] It can be difficult to clinically and neuropathologically differentiate between PD with dementia and DLB, and it remains controversial whether these are two completely different neurological diseases or just two presentations within the spectrum of Lewy body diseases.

Clinical characteristics

DLB should be suspected in patients with mild parkinsonism who demonstrate progressive cognitive decline, fluctuating levels of alertness, and visual and/or auditory hallucinations. These symptoms may also be accompanied by executive dysfunction, memory loss, aphasia, and visuospatial disorientation. In 1996, consensus criteria for the diagnosis of DLB were developed (Table 3.4).[16] In 1999, the report of the second DLB international workshop suggested that depression and rapid eye movement sleep behavior disorder were additional supportive features.

Ancillary tests

There are no consistent MRI findings characteristic of DLB, but neuropsychological testing can be helpful toward better defining the cognitive deficits.

Corticobasal degeneration

Epidemiology

CBD is a rare neurodegenerative disease that was first described by Rebeiz et al.[17] in 1968. The incidence and prevalence of CBD is unknown and is probably underestimated. This is further complicated by the fact that more

Table 3.4 Consensus criteria for the clinical diagnosis of probable and possible dementia with Lewy bodies

Diagnostic categories	Inclusion criteria	Exclusion criteria	Supportive criteria
Possible	Progressive cognitive decline of sufficient magnitude to interfere with normal social or occupational function. Prominent or persistent memory impairment may not necessarily occur in the early stages but is usually evident with progression. Deficits on tests of attention and of frontal-subcortical skills and visuospatial ability may be especially prominent. One of three core features: (1) fluctuating cognition with pronounced variations in attention and alertness, (2) recurrent visual hallucinations, (3) parkinsonism	For possible and probable: stroke disease or evidence of any other brain disorder sufficient to account for the clinical picture	Repeated falls, syncope, transient loss of consciousness, neuroleptic sensitivity, systematized delusions, hallucinations in other modalities[a]
Probable	Possible criteria plus one core feature		
Definite	Autopsy confirmation		

[a] Depression and rapid eye movement sleep behavior disorder have since been suggested as additional supportive features.

Source: Litvan I, Bhatia KP, Burn DJ, et al. Movement Disorders Society Scientific Issues Committee report: SIC Task Force appraisal of clinical diagnostic criteria for Parkinsonian disorders. *Mov Disord.* 2003;18(5):467–486. Reprinted with permission.

than one entity can present with features originally ascribed to CBD. Therefore, many refer to *corticobasal syndrome*, recognizing that CBD is one pathological cause of this syndrome. CBD is a sporadic disorder presenting in mid- to late adult life (mean age of onset 63 years) and leading to death approximately 5 to 10 years after symptom onset. Shorter length of survival has been found to be associated with early onset of bilateral parkinsonism and frontal dysfunction.

Clinical characteristics
CBD typically presents with unilateral limb (typically the arm) clumsiness, stiffness, jerking, or sensory abnormality. The limb may be held in a fixed dystonic posture. Over the course of the disease, patients may also develop rigidity, focal reflex myoclonus, and a postural and action tremor. The typical parkinsonian resting tremor is not a feature of CBD.

Frequently, apraxia is noted, especially ideomotor and limb-kinetic apraxia; however, it can be especially difficult to differentiate the latter from clumsiness secondary to extrapyramidal dysfunction. Some patients develop alien-limb phenomenon and cortical sensory deficits. Over years the disease progresses to affect other limbs, and eventually becomes a bilateral phenomenon. In time, the combination of apraxia, dystonia, rigidity, akinesia, and myoclonus can make the affected limbs functionally useless. One characteristic feature of CBD, which is similar to the other atypical parkinsonian syndromes, is that the motor symptoms have poor or no response to levodopa treatment. In advanced stages there also may be oculomotor abnormalities. However, in contrast to PSP, these are equally severe in the vertical and horizontal directions, and saccadic latencies are more impaired than velocities. Initially, there is usually no evidence of cognitive deterioration or dysphasia; however, these features can develop later. Rarely, patients present with dementia or an abnormal neuropsychological profile prior to developing motor deficits. The neuropsychiatric abnormalities that can be seen in CBD include depression, apathy, anxiety, irritability, disinhibition, and obsessive-compulsive disorder. While there are published criteria for the diagnosis of CBD, none have been formally validated. At this time, as with the other atypical parkinsonian syndromes, ultimate diagnosis is based on neuropathology in conjunction with the clinical picture.

Ancillary tests

In the early stages of the CBD, MRI brain images are typically normal. However, as the disease progresses, CBD is characterized by asymmetrical atrophy in the posterior frontal and parietal cortices, often contralateral to the side of the clinical manifestations.

Summary

While PD is the most common cause of parkinsonism, there are other disease processes that should be considered in the differential diagnosis of PD. Through careful history taking and physical examination, one may be able to elicit some atypical features that might point to another parkinsonian syndrome. The currently accepted diagnostic criteria for PSP, MSA, and DLB, in conjunction with appropriate ancillary testing, should be helpful in making the correct diagnosis, which is crucial as better therapeutic options are developed.

References

1. Hughes AJ, Daniel SE, Kilford L, Lees AJ. Accuracy of clinical diagnosis of idiopathic Parkinson's disease: a clinico-pathological study of 100 cases. *J Neurol Neurosurg Psychiatry*. 1992;55:181–184.

2. Wenning GK, Ebersbach G, Verny M, et al. Progression of falls in postmortem-confirmed parkinsonian disorders. *Mov Disord*. 1999;14:947–950.

3. Giladi N, Burke RE, Kostic V, et al. Hemiparkinsonism-hemiatrophy syndrome: clinical and neuroradiologic features. *Neurology*. 1990;40:1731–1734.

4. Wenning GK, Scherfler C, Granata R, et al. Time course of symptomatic orthostatic hypotension and urinary incontinence in patients with postmortem confirmed parkinsonian syndromes: a clinicopathological study. *J Neurol Neurosurg Psychiatry*. 1999;67:620–623.

5. Rivaud-Pechoux S, Vidailhet M, Gallouedec G, Litvan I, Gaymard B, Pierrot-Deseilligny C. Longitudinal ocular motor study in corticobasal degeneration and progressive supranuclear palsy. *Neurology*. 2000;54:1029–1032.

6. Merello M, Nouzeilles MI, Arce GP, Leiguarda R. Accuracy of acute levodopa challenge for clinical prediction of sustained long-term levodopa response as a major criterion for idiopathic Parkinson's disease diagnosis. *Mov Disord*. 2002;17:795–798.

7. Nath U, Ben-Shlomo Y, Thomson RG, et al. The prevalence of progressive supranuclear palsy (Steele-Richardson-Olszewski syndrome) in the UK. *Brain*. 2001;124:1438–1449.

8. Schrag A, Ben-Shlomo Y, Quinn NP. Prevalence of progressive supra-nuclear palsy and multiple system atrophy: a cross-sectional study. *Lancet*. 1999;354:1771–1775.

9. Golbe LI, Davis PH, Schoenberg BS, Duvoisin RC. Prevalence and natural history of progressive supranuclear palsy. *Neurology*. 1988;38:1031–1034.

10. Ben-Shlomo Y, Wenning GK, Tison F, Quinn NP. Survival of patients with pathologically proven multiple system atrophy: a meta-analysis. *Neurology*. 1997;48:384–393.

11. Schwarz J, Weis S, Kraft E, et al. Signal changes on MRI and increases in reactive microgliosis, astrogliosis, and iron in the putamen of two patients with multiple system atrophy. *J Neurol Neurosurg Psychiatry*. 1996;60:98–101.

12. Schocke MF, Seppi K, Esterhammer R, et al. Diffusion-weighted MRI differentiates the Parkinson variant of multiple system atrophy from PD. *Neurology*. 2002;58:575–580.

13. Vodusek DB. Sphincter EMG and differential diagnosis of multiple system atrophy. *Mov Disord*. 2001;16:600–607.

14. McKeith IG, Galasko D, Kosaka K, et al. Consensus guidelines for the clinical and pathologic diagnosis of dementia with Lewy bodies (DLB): report of the consortium on DLB international workshop. *Neurology*. 1996;47:1113–1124.

15. Aarsland D, Andersen K, Larsen JP, Lolk A, Nielsen H, Kragh-Sorensen P. Risk of dementia in Parkinson's disease: a community-based, prospective study. *Neurology*. 2001;56:730–736.

16. Rebeiz JJ, Kolodny EH, Richardson EP Jr. Corticodentatonigral degeneration with neuronal achromasia. *Arch Neurol*. 1968;18:20–33.

Chapter 4

The role of imaging in the diagnosis and differential diagnosis of Parkinson's disease

Danna Jennings

Parkinson's disease (PD) is a progressive condition diagnosed by the cardinal clinical features of resting tremor, rigidity, and bradykinesia. While the diagnosis in many cases is easily recognized, the variability of disease presentation or an unclear response to therapy can make the diagnosis uncertain. Long-term clinicopathologic studies evaluating the diagnostic accuracy of PD demonstrate error rates of up to 24%. The diagnoses most commonly mistaken for PD are progressive supranuclear palsy (PSP) and multiple system atrophy (MSA).[1–3] However, early in the course of PD the diagnoses most commonly mistaken for PD include essential tremor (ET), vascular parkinsonism, drug-induced parkinsonism, and Alzheimer's disease.[4,5]

Neuroimaging has provided key insights into the natural history of PD and has emerged as an important diagnostic tool. The two primary approaches to imaging are structural, using magnetic resonance imaging (MRI), and functional radiotracer imaging, using either single photon emission computerized tomography (SPECT) or photon emission tomography (PET). SPECT and PET imaging use specific radioactively labeled ligands to neurochemically tag or mark normal or abnormal brain chemistry. Recent advances in radioligand development and imaging technologies have expanded the role of imaging in PD. Recent developments in MRI techniques are also useful in the differential diagnosis of PD.

Imaging methodology

The main pathological finding in PD is degeneration of presynaptic dopaminergic cells projecting from the substantia nigra to the striatum (caudate and putamen). The integrity of the presynaptic dopaminergic system can be assessed using radiotracer imaging in conjunction with SPECT or PET imaging. The imaging ligands ^{18}F-DOPA, ^{11}C-VMAT2, and dopamine transporter (DAT) ligands target different components of the presynaptic nigrostriatal neuron. Properties of each these targets are outlined in Table 4.1. The most widely studied tracers for PD include the DAT ligands

Table 4.1 Comparison of dopamine presynaptic ligands in Parkinson's disease studies

	[¹²³I]β-CIT	¹¹C-VMAT2	¹⁸F-DOPA
Target	DA transporter	Vesicular transporter	DA turnover
Bilateral reduction in hemi-PD	Yes	Yes	Yes
Correlates with UPDRS in cross section	Yes	Yes	Yes
Annual reduction change with aging (% loss from baseline)	0.8% to 1.4%	0.5%	None

DA, dopamine. PD, Parkinson's disease. UPDRS, Unified Parkinson Disease Rating Scale.

[¹²³I]β-CIT and [¹²³I]FP-CIT. While none of the tracers is currently commercially available in North America, ¹²³FP-CIT (DaTSCAN) is available in Europe. Numerous clinical imaging studies have shown an asymmetrical reduction in ¹⁸F-DOPA, ¹¹C-VMAT2, and DAT ligand uptake in PD.[6–8]

Imaging as a diagnostic tool in PD

Routine structural MRI has limited value and is not necessary in the diagnosis of PD. While MRI imaging in advanced cases can demonstrate atrophy of the substantia nigra, the findings are not reproducible and are not particularly useful for diagnostic purposes. PET and SPECT ligands have been shown to differentiate clinically probable PD patients from normal subjects or patients with ET cases with approximately 90% sensitivity and specificity.[9–11] This makes imaging a valuable diagnostic tool in PD. The reduction in DAT ligand uptake in PD is more pronounced in the putamen, with relative sparing of the caudate in the early stages of the disease (Fig. 4.1). These imaging findings are consistent with both pathological assessment of the DAT loss and clinical presentation of PD. In studies focused on early PD patients, at the threshold of illness DAT imaging demonstrated a 40% to 60% reduction in DAT or F-DOPA activity in the putamen, with changes that were asymmetrical and more pronounced contralateral to the symptomatic side.

In general, PD initially presents as a unilateral motor disorder and progresses during a variable period of 3 to 6 years to affect both sides, although frequently remaining asymmetrical. The unilateral motor presentation reflects the asymmetrical dopaminergic pathology, which is in turn demonstrated by in vivo dopaminergic imaging.[9,12] While DAT imaging is considered to be a useful tool in differentiating parkinsonism without dopaminergic degeneration, it is less applicable in differentiating atypical parkinsonism (Fig. 4.2).

Interestingly, when specific PD symptoms are compared, the loss of dopaminergic activity measured by imaging correlates with bradykinesia

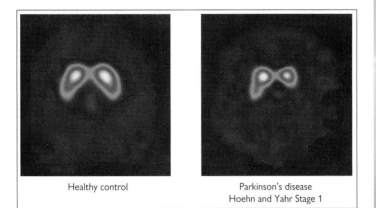

| Healthy control | Parkinson's disease |
| | Hoehn and Yahr Stage 1 |

Figure 4.1 Dopamine transporter imaging using [^{123}I]β-CIT SPECT in a healthy control and a Parkinson's disease (PD) subject. There is reduction in the uptake of [^{123}I]β -CIT in the putamen in the PD subject.

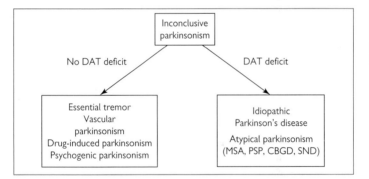

Figure 4.2 Dopamine transporter imaging as a tool for differentiating conditions with a presynaptic dopaminergic degeneration recognized as a DAT deficit by imaging.

but not with tremor.[10,13] Cross-sectional studies show that severity of bradykinesia measured by clinical scales reflects the severity of the nigrostriatal dopamine neuron loss. This suggests that in vivo dopaminergic imaging is also a marker for disease severity.

Making an accurate diagnosis of PD is most difficult early in the course, at the threshold of symptoms. DAT imaging studies involving patients with suspected parkinsonian syndrome have been performed to determine the sensitivity and specificity of DAT imaging as a diagnostic tool in this difficult-to-diagnose population. In these studies, the baseline DAT imaging diagnosis was compared to 6- to 12-month clinical follow-up by a movement disorder expert masked to the imaging data, which was considered to be the gold standard diagnosis. The sensitivity of the [^{123}I]β-CIT SPECT imaging diagnosis was 90% to 92% and specificity 89% to 100% when compared to the clinical gold standard diagnosis.[14,15] For subjects in whom the imaging and clinical diagnoses remained incongruent, possible diagnoses included ET, lower-body parkinsonism likely of vascular etiology, and drug-induced parkinsonism. A similar study was conducted utilizing [^{123}I]FP-CIT SPECT. The subjects were followed over a period of 2 to 4 years. The clinicians were aware of the imaging results and utilized this information in making a final diagnosis. In 9 out of 33 subjects, there was imaging evidence of presynaptic dopaminergic neuronal degeneration, and in all cases a diagnosis of parkinsonian syndrome was confirmed clinically. In 24 subjects there was no imaging evidence of dopaminergic neuronal degeneration, and other nonparkinsonian diagnoses were assigned in 19 of these subjects at follow-up. In two cases the clinical diagnosis of presynaptic parkinsonism was retained despite normal imaging data.[16] These studies suggest a high positive predictive value for DAT imaging in the diagnosis of presynaptic parkinsonism. DAT imaging provides a valuable addition to the clinical evaluation and appears to be the most useful at the threshold of illness, when the diagnosis remains uncertain.

While accurately diagnosing individuals early in the course of PD clearly impacts the clinical care of individuals, it may also have implications for early PD clinical trials. Two recent studies using [^{123}I]β-CIT SPECT and ^{18}F-dopa PET as surrogate markers have found that about 6% to 14% of individuals with the diagnosis of early PD who were enrolled in these studies had no evidence of reduced tracer uptake. They were labeled as symptomatic without evidence of dopaminergic deficit (SWEDD).[17,18] In the Requip as Early Therapy versus L-dopa PET (REAL-PET) study, which compared ropinirole and levodopa as initial treatments in patients with early untreated PD, 11% (21/193) of enrolled subjects were classified as SWEDD at baseline and after two years. In the Earlier versus Later L-dopa (ELLDOPA) trial, which compared initial levodopa therapy to placebo in recently diagnosed PD patients, 14% (21/142) of enrolled subjects were SWEDD at baseline. Possible explanations for the inconsistency between the clinical and imaging diagnoses are that the SWEDD subjects were clinically misdiagnosed or that DAT imaging is not a sensitive measure of changes early in the course of disease. Evidence is now available to suggest that SWEDD subjects most likely have conditions not affecting the nigrostriatal dopaminergic pathway. Studies have shown a strong correlation between DAT uptake on SPECT and the levels of striatal dopamine.[19,20]

Provided that approximately 50% of dopaminergic neurons have degenerated by the time of symptom onset, it is unlikely that DAT imaging would not be able to detect this degree of loss. Follow-up of SWEDD subjects has shown that there is no change in SWEDD status on repeat imaging. In the ELLDOPA study, 19 out of 19 remained SWEDD at 9-month follow-up, and in the REAL-PET study 21 of 21 remained SWEDD at 2 years. The data from these studies suggest that SWEDD subjects most likely have conditions that do not affect the nigrostriatal dopaminergic pathway.

Differentiating PD from ET

ET is characterized by the presence of bilateral postural and action tremor of the upper limbs or head. While the diagnosis of ET is usually straightforward, diagnostic difficulties can arise when there also appears to be a rest component to the tremor, associated cogwheel rigidity (which can commonly occur in ET), or asymmetry of symptoms. Patients with classic ET without overlapping features have DAT imaging in the range expected for age. Studies investigating the potential of DAT imaging to differentiate ET from PD have found a sensitivity and specificity of about 95% of DAT and SPECT for successfully discriminating between the two disorders.[11,21] DAT and SPECT imaging reliably distinguish between individuals with PD or other parkinsonian syndromes and ET.

Differentiating PD from drug-induced parkinsonism

Parkinsonism related to antidopaminergic drug exposure is common in older patients and in populations with psychiatric disorders. Postsynaptic dopamine-receptor blocking agents, primarily antipsychotics and centrally acting antiemetics, are the most frequent offending medications in drug-induced parkinsonism. Withdrawal of dopamine-receptor blocking medication can require several months to reach full resolution of parkinsonian symptoms. Differentiating drug-induced parkinsonism from a parkinsonian syndrome with nigrostriatal degeneration can be difficult clinically, but it has significant implications for treatment and prognosis.

Evaluating the integrity of the presynaptic dopamine neurons using DAT imaging provides valuable diagnostic information in cases suspected to be drug-induced. While there are few reports of patients with drug-induced parkinsonism undergoing DAT imaging, [^{123}I]FP-CIT was found to be in the normal range in three drug-induced cases,[16] and one subject with drug-induced parkinsonism (based on follow-up clinical examination) had normal age-expected uptake of [^{123}I]β –CIT.[14] While the data are limited, DAT imaging appears to be a useful tool in differentiating parkinsonism caused by dopamine-receptor blocking agents from parkinsonism due to striatonigral dopaminergic neuronal loss.

Differentiating PD from vascular parkinsonism

Vascular parkinsonism is a poorly defined syndrome. Diagnostic questions often arise when a patient presents with parkinsonism and diffuse white matter ischemic changes or lacunar lesions localized to the basal ganglia. Vascular parkinsonism typically presents with no tremor and symptoms of rigidity and bradykinesia predominantly in the lower extremities, which results in a gait disorder and postural instability. This syndrome is frequently referred to as lower-body parkinsonism.

While in a majority of cases this syndrome is believed to be of vascular etiology and is levodopa-resistant, some patients with idiopathic PD, specifically those at an older age at onset, can have similar presentation, which makes the differential diagnosis a challenge. Pathological studies have shown preservation of the presynaptic dopaminergic circuitry in vascular parkinsonism patients.[22,23] It has been hypothesized that deep periventricular white-matter lesions disrupt connections between the primary motor cortex and the supplementary motor cortex with the cerebellum and the basal ganglia. A definitive diagnosis of vascular parkinsonism requires neuropathologic evaluation postmortem. However, at least one study of 13 subjects who fulfilled the criteria for a clinical diagnosis of vascular parkinsonism demonstrated preservation of DAT uptake with [123I]β-CIT and SPECT imaging.[24]

In another series of 20 patients with cerebrovascular changes and parkinsonism, more than half showed a reduction in [123I]FP-CIT.[25] All subjects with normal DAT uptake had no response to levodopa. Among the 11 subjects with abnormal DAT uptake, half were levodopa responsive. In conclusion, while DAT imaging may not provide a definitive differentiation in all cases, a diagnosis of vascular parkinsonism can be made in cases with vascular lesions and normal DAT imaging.

Differentiating PD from psychogenic parkinsonism

Psychogenic parkinsonism is a rare syndrome responsible for less than 10% of all cases of psychogenic movement disorders. Studies have shown that 10% to 25% of patients with psychogenic movement disorders had features of both organic and psychogenic disorders.[26,27] Experts often need to follow an individual patient over a period of time to definitively differentiate psychogenic parkinsonism from PD. In cases with a clear clinical diagnosis of psychogenic parkinsonism, there is no evidence of dopaminergic neuronal degeneration. Using DAT imaging in cases of suspected psychogenic parkinsonism provides additional objective information to help differentiate from a parkinsonian syndrome related to nigrostriatal dopaminergic degeneration. There are limited reports in which a few patients with suspected psychogenic parkinsonsim have undergone DAT imaging. In a study of 33 subjects with suspected parkinsonism, 19 had normal [123I]FP-CIT, four of whom were ultimately diagnosed with psychogenic parkinsonism.[16] In a separate series, two patients with a final clinical diagnosis of psychogenic parkinsonism had [123I]β -CIT scans in the normal range expected for their age.[14] These reports suggest that normal DAT imaging can be useful as supportive data in the diagnosis of psychogenic parkinsonism.

Differentiating Parkinson's disease from atypical parkinsonian disorders

The most common etiology of parkinsonian syndrome is PD, while atypical parkinsonian disorders account for about 15% to 20% of parkinsonian patients. The most common atypical parkinsonian syndromes are progressive supranuclear palsy (PSP), multiple systems atrophy (MSA), and corticobasal degeneration (CBD). The clinical differential diagnosis of these syndromes is discussed in Chapter 3. Routine MRI has been shown to be valuable in differentiating PD from atypical parkinsonian disorders.[28,29] Structural and volumetric MRI changes described in MSA include atrophy of the medulla, pons, and cerebellum and hyperintensity of the middle cerebellar peduncle, cerebellum, inferior olives, and pons, resulting in the "hot cross bun" sign. The MRI changes recognized in PSP include midbrain atrophy, globus pallidus hyperintesity, and fronto-temporal cortical atrophy. While these structural MRI changes have been reported to be highly specific, the sensitivity of these changes is less than 60% to 80%. More recently, diffusion-weighted imaging (DWI) has been developed and has the potential to be useful in differentiating PD from atypical parkinsonian disorders.[30] DWI relies on measurement of movement of water molecules through the fiber tracts of the nervous system. Water molecules mainly move along the fiber tracts in nervous tissue, and neurodegeneration appears to increase water-molecule mobility, resulting in increased diffusion. Recent studies have suggested that DWI can distinguish MSA and PSP from PD with high sensitivity within a few years from disease onset.[31] However, DWI does not appear to be a reliable way to distinguish MSA from PSP. Summary of the MRI findings in parkinsonian syndromes is presented in Table 4.2.

Table 4.2 MRI findings in parkinsonian syndromes

Parkinson's disease

T2-weighted MRI: essentially normal

May possibly see (later in the disease course):

- Hypointense putamen > pallidum
- Hypointense posterolateral putamen
- Decreased width in substantia nigra pars compacta

MR volumetry: normal

DWI: normal

Multiple systems atrophy

Atrophy

- Putamen
- Pons
- Middle cerebellar peduncle
- Cerebellum

T2-weighted fast spin sequences

- Hypointense putamen
- Hyperintense lateral putaminal rim
- Hot cross bun sign
- Hyperintense middle cerebellar peduncle
- Cerebellar hyperintensities

T2-weighted gradient echo sequences

- Hypointense putamen

DWI

- Increased putaminal rADC

Progressive supranuclear palsy

T2-weighted MRI

- Midbrain atrophy, anteroposterior (AP) diameter < 17 mm
- Midsagittal hummingbird sign
- Enlarged third ventricle (due to atrophy) with:
  - Flattening of quadrigeminal plate
  - Slight periaqueductal hyperintensity
  - Thinning of the tectal plate

Table 4.2 *continued*
DWI
* Increased ADC in putamen, caudate, pallidum
Volumetry
Midbrain and frontal volume loss
Corticobasal syndrome
* Asymmetrical cortical atrophy
* Posterior frontal cortex atrophy
* Superior parietal cortex atrophy
* Atrophy of the middle portion of corpus callosum
T1-weighted MRI
* Hypointense signal change in putamen
T2-weighted MRI
* Hyperintense signal change in the motor cortex and SCWM

ADC, apparent diffusion coefficient; DWI, diffusion-weighted imaging; MRI, magnetic resonance imaging; rADC, regional ADC; RN, red nucleus; SCWM, subcortical white matter; SNC, substantia nigra pars compacta; SNR, substantia nigra pars reticulata.

Functional imaging also has a role in the differential diagnosis of parkinsonian syndromes. The presynaptic dopaminergic loss is demonstrated by reduction of in vivo presynaptic dopaminergic imaging. While the severity of DAT or ^{18}F-DOPA loss does not discriminate between PD and atypical parkinsonian disorders, the pattern of loss in the latter is less region-specific (putamen and caudate equally affected) and more symmetrical than in PD. This strategy discriminates between PD and atypical parkinsonian disorders with a sensitivity of about 75% to 80%.[32,33] In addition, the more widespread pathology associated with atypical parkinsonian disorders may be reflected in abnormalities in postsynaptic dopamine receptor imaging and metabolic imaging that are not seen in PD. Therefore the pattern of presynaptic dopaminergic loss may be coupled with postsynaptic dopamine receptor imaging or metabolic imaging to distinguish PD from other related parkinsonian syndromes.[34,35]

Imaging to detect preclinical Parkinson's disease

Imaging studies of the presynaptic dopaminergic terminals provide a window into the preclinical period of PD, the time during which neurodegeneration has begun but symptoms have not yet become manifest. Data from longitudinal imaging studies using both [18F]DOPA and DAT imaging have estimated a preclinical phase of 4 to 8 years.[17,36] The most extensive preclinical imaging data are from studies that imaged patients with hemi-PD. The data show a significant reduction in putamen DAT or [18F]DOPA uptake of about 25% to 30% in the presymptomatic striatum in these patients, who are known to progress to bilateral disease.[12] Some studies of the preclinical period have focused on potential at-risk individuals for PD, such as family members or unaffected twins of PD patients. A recent study that evaluated hyposmic first-degree relatives of PD patients showed that

4 out of 40 (10%) hyposmic relatives with no parkinsonian signs converted to PD over a 2-year period.[37] Of the 40 subjects, 7 showed a reduction in [^{123}I]β-CIT uptake, and the 4 with the lowest uptake were those converting to PD. Findings from this study suggest that DAT imaging has the capacity to detect changes in the DAT prior to the onset of symptoms, thus serving as a preclinical marker. Moving toward preclinical identification of PD may provide the opportunity to intervene at an earlier stage of disease and may offer the possibility of delaying or even preventing the onset of symptoms once neuroprotective treatment strategies are developed.

While dopaminergic neuronal degeneration is a primary pathological feature of PD, it is clear that there is widespread degeneration in the brain in PD. It becoming more widely recognized that many of the clinical manifestations of PD are likely not exclusively associated with dopaminergic neuronal loss. Evidence suggests that PD pathological changes may begin in the lower brain-stem nuclei, predating changes in the dopaminergic neurons. Ligands for nondopaminergic targets, including noradrenergic cells in the locus ceruleus, serotonergic cells in the median raphae, and inflammatory markers of microglial activation, are under development to investigate nondopaminergic manifestations of PD and to better understand the pathophysiology of PD. The role of brain imaging in PD will continue to expand as new imaging targets emerge and disease-modifying drugs are developed. As additional genetic and screening tools to identify preclinical at-risk individuals become available, neuroreceptor imaging will be widely used to establish and monitor the natural history of the preclinical stage and the onset of disease.

References

1. Rajput A, Rodzilsky B, Rajput A. Accuracy of clinical diagnosis of Parkinsonism—a prospective study. *Can J Neurol Sci*. 1991;18:275–278.

2. Hughes AJ, Daniel SE, Kilford L, Lees AJ. Accuracy of clinical diagnosis of idiopathic Parkinson's disease: a clinico-pathological study of 100 cases. *J Neurol Neurosurg Psychiatry*. 1992;55:1142–1146.

3. Hughes AJ, Daniel SE, Ben-Shlomo Y, Lees AJ. The accuracy of diagnosis of parkinsonian syndromes in a specialist movement disorder service. *Brain*. 2002;125:861–870.

4. Quinn N. Parkinsonism—recognition and differential diagnosis. *BMJ*. 1995;310:447–452.

5. Meara J, Bhowmick BK, Hobson P. Accuracy of diagnosis in patients with presumed Parkinson's disease. *Age and Ageing*. 1999;28:99–102.

6. Brooks DJ. Positron emission tomography studies in movement disorders. *Neurosurg Clin N Am*. 1998;9:263–282.

7. Marek K. Dopaminergic dysfunction in Parkinsonism: new lessons from imaging. *Neuroscientist*. 1999;5:333–339.

8. Frey K, Koeppe R, Kilbourn M. Imaging the vesicular monoamine transporter. *Adv Neurol*. 2001;86:237–247.

9. Sawle G, Playford E, Burn D, Cunnigham V, Brooks D. Separating Parkinson's disease from normality: discriminant function analysis of [18F]dopa PET data. *Arch Neurol*. 1994;51:237–243.

10. Seibyl JP, Marek KL, Quinlan D, et al. Decreased single-photon emission computed tomographic [¹²³I]β -CIT striatal uptake correlates with symptom severity in Parkinson's disease. *Ann Neurol.* 1995;38:589–598.

11. Benamer TS, Patterson J, Grosset DG, et al. Accurate differentiation of parkinsonism and essential tremor using visual assessment of [¹²³I]-FP-CIT SPECT imaging: the [¹²³I]-FP CIT study group. *Mov Disord.* 2000;15:503–510.

12. Marek K, Seibyl J, Scanley B, et al. [¹²³I]β-CIT SPECT imaging demonstrates bilateral loss of dopamine transporters in hemi Parkinson's disease. *Neurology.* 1996;46:231–237.

13. Vingerhoets FJ, Schulzer M, Calne DB, Snow BJ. Which clinical sign of Parkinson's disease best reflects the nigrostriatal lesion? *Ann Neurol.* 1997;41:58–64.

14. Jennings DJ, Seibyl JP, Oakes D, Eberly S, Murphy J, Marek K. [¹²³I]β-CIT and SPECT imaging versus clinical evaluation in parkinsonian syndrome: unmasking an early diagnosis. *Arch Neurol.* 2004;61:1224–1229.

15. Jennings DL, Tabamo R, Seibyl JP, Marek K. Evaluation of dopamine transporter imaging as a tool for the early diagnosis of parkinsonian syndromes. *Neurology.* 2005;64(6 suppl):A253.

16. Booij J, Speelman JD, Horstink MW, Wolters EC. The clinical benefit of imaging striatal dopamine transporter with [¹²³I]FP-CIT SPET in differentiating patients with presynaptic parkinsonism from those with other forms of parkinsonism. *Eur J Nucl Med.* 2001;28(3):266–72.

17. Fahn S, Parkinson Study Group. Does levodopa slow or hasten the rate of progression of Parkinson's disease? *J Neurol.* 2005;2524(suppl):37–42.

18. Whone A, Remy P, Davis MR, et al. The REAL-PET study: slower progression in early Parkinson's disease treated with ropinirole compared with L-Dopa. *Neurology.* 2002;58(suppl 13):A82–A83.

19. Bezard E, Dovero S, Prunier C, et al. Relationship between the appearance of symptoms and the level of nigrostriatal degeneration in a progressive 1-methyl-4-phenyl-1,2,3,6 tetrahydropyridine-lesioned macaque model of Parkinson's disease. *J Neurosci.* 2001;21:6853–6861.

20. Porritt M, Stanic D, Finkelstein D, et al. Dopaminergic innervation of the human striatum in Parkinson's disease. *Mov Disord.* 2005;20:810–818.

21. Asenbaum S, Pirker W, Angelberger P, Bencsits G, Pruckmayer M, Brucke T. [¹²³I]β-CIT and SPECT in essential tremor and Parkinson's disease. *J Neural Transm.* 1998;105:1213–1228.

22. Jellinger KA. Parkinsonism due to Binswanger's subcortical arteriosclerotic encephalopathy. *Mov Disord.* 1996;11:461–462.

23. Yamanouchi H, Nagura H. Neurological signs and frontal white matter lesions in vascular parkinsonism. *Stroke.* 1997;28:965–969.

24. Gerschlager W, Bencsits G, Pirker W, et al. [¹²³I]β-CIT SPECT distinguishes vascular parkinsonism from Parkinson's disease. *Mov Disord.* 2002;17(3):518–523.

25. Lorberboyn M, Djaldetti R, Melamed E, Sadeh M, Lampl Y. [¹²³I]FP-CIT SPECT imaging of dopamine transporters in patients with cerebrovascular disease and a clinical diagnosis of vascular parkinsonism. *J Nucl Med.* 2004;45:1688–1693.

26. Ranawaya R, Riley D, Lang A. Psychogenic dyskinesias in patients with organic movement disorders. *Mov Disord.* 1990;5(2):127–133.

27. Factor SA, Podskalny GD, Molho ES. Psychogenic movement disorders: frequency, clinical profile, characteristics. *J Neurol Neurosurg Psychiatry.* 1995;59:406–412.

28. Schrag A, Good CD, Miszkiel K, et al. Differentiation of atypical parkinsonian syndromes with routine MRI. *Neurology.* 2000;54:607–702.

29. Kraft E, Trenkwalder C, Auer DP. T2-weighted MRI differentiates multiple systems atrophy from Parkinson's disease. *Neurology.* 2002;59:1265–1267.

30. Schocke M, Seppi K, Esterhammer R, et al. Diffusion weighted MRI differentiates the Parkinson variant of multiple systems atrophy from PD. *Neurology.* 2002;58:575–580.

31. Seppi K, Schoecke MF, Esterhammer R, et al. Diffusion-weighted imaging discriminates progressive supranuclear palsy from PD, but not from the Parkinson variant of multiple system atrophy. *Neurology.* 2003;60:922–927.

32. Brucke T, Asenbaum S, Pirker W, et al. Measurement of the dopaminergic degeneration in Parkinson's disease with [^{123}I]β-CIT and SPECT. Correlation with clinical findings and comparison with multiple system atrophy and progressive supranuclear palsy. *J Neural Transm Suppl.* 1997;50:9–24.

33. Varrone A, Marek KL, Jennings D, Innis RB, and Seibyl JP. [^{123}I]β-CIT SPECT imaging demonstrates reduced density of striatal dopamine transporters in Parkinson's disease and multiple system atrophy. *Mov Disord.* 2001;16:1023–1032.

34. Antonini A, Kazumata K, Feigin A, et al. Differential diagnosis of parkinsonism with [18F]fluorodeoxyglucose and PET. *Mov Disord.* 1998;13:268–274.

35. Eidelberg D, Dhawan V. Can imaging distinguish PSP from other neurodegenerative disorders? *Neurology.* 2002;58:997–998.

36. Morrish P, Rakshi J, Bailey D, Sawle G, Brooks D. Measuring the rate of progression and estimating the preclinical period of Parkinson's disease with [18F]dopa PET. *J Neurol Neurosurg Psychiatry.* 1998;64:314–319.

37. Ponsen MM, Stoffers D, Booij J, van Eck-Smit B, Wolters EC, Berendse HW. Idiopathic hyposmia as a preclinical sign of Parkinson's disease. *Ann Neurol.* 2004;56:173–181.

Chapter 5

Etiology of Parkinson's disease

Arif Dalvi and Ryan Walsh

Sir James Parkinson considered "indulgence in spirituous liquors" and "long lying on the damp ground" as possible etiologies of Parkinson's disease (PD).[1] Eighty years later, Gower reported that 15% of his patients with PD had a family history.[2] More recently, initial impressions from a twin study on World War II veterans suggested a minor role for genetic factors, as similar concordance rates were observed in monozygotic and dizygotic twins.[3] However, following the discovery of the α-synuclein gene[4] and the subsequent discovery of a number of PARK genes, the debate between supporters of genetic or environmental causes has been renewed. The assumptions of Sir James Parkinson have not held up, but a number of alternative environmental factors have been brought into the limelight. This review is focused on "idiopathic" PD, although causes of atypical parkinsonism are reviewed where they offer relevant insights. Current understanding of the etiology of PD points to a multifactorial disorder with gene–environment interactions leading to neuronal cell death (Fig. 5.1).

Selective vulnerability of the dopaminergic system

The selective vulnerability of the substantia nigra pars compacta (SNc) in the pathogenesis of PD is an area of active study. There are several leading hypotheses, and it is likely a combination of these that explains SNc vulnerability. First, oxidative stress involving mitochondrial dysfunction may be over-represented in SNc, primarily due to reactive oxidation species produced during dopamine storage and breakdown. Models of endoplasmic reticulum stress show age-dependent selective vulnerability of dopaminergic neurons, also related to the oxidative byproducts of dopamine metabolism.[5] Dopamine metabolites, especially the monoamine oxidase metabolite 3,4-dihydroxyphenylacetaldehyde, can trigger α-synuclein aggregation in SNc neurons. The unique susceptibility of the long axons of SNc to microtubule dysfunction may result in accumulation of cytosolic dopamine, leading to oxidative stress. Furthermore, deficiencies in the structure and function of the ubiquitin/proteasome system have been identified in SNc of PD patients,[6] and levels of proteasome activators important

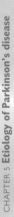

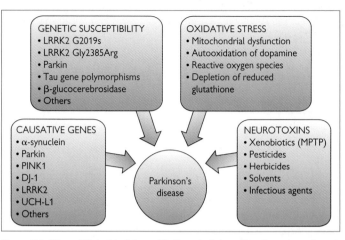

Figure 5.1 The multifactorial etiology of Parkinson's disease. Causative genes and genetic susceptibility factors interact with environmental triggers and endogenous causes of oxidative stress. Misfolding and aggregation of proteins together with mitochondrial dysfunction provide the framework for neuronal cell death leading to Parkinson's disease. © Arif Dalvi, 2007.

for normal function of this system are altered in SNc more than other brain regions.[7] Finally, SNc may be particularly vulnerable to the dysfunction of micro-RNAs possibly involved in maintenance of dopaminergic neurons.[8] Importantly, the five genes currently linked with familial PD are, to varying degrees, implicated in the function and dysfunction of the cellular processes listed earlier, and represent possible contributors to the selective vulnerability of SNc in PD.

The discovery of the α-synuclein gene was followed by the observation that it is a significant component of Lewy bodies, which are the pathological hallmark of PD. The mechanism whereby mutant α-synuclein causes PD remains to be defined. Learning how mutant α-synuclein causes PD is also relevant to sporadic PD, as dopaminergic neurons in these cases also show Lewy bodies rich in α-synuclein. Wild-type α-synuclein is selectively translocated into lysosomes for degradation by the chaperone-mediated autophagy pathway. The pathogenic A53T and A30P variants bind to a transporter within lysosomes inside the dopaminergic neurons. Once bound, they appear to act as uptake blockers, inhibiting both their own degradation and that of other substrates. As a consequence, toxic proteins build up inside neurons, leading eventually to neuronal death.[9]

Accumulation of α-synuclein in cultured human dopaminergic neurons has been shown to result in apoptotic cell death. This mechanism requires endogenous dopamine production and is mediated by reactive oxygen species. In contrast, α-synuclein is neuroprotective in nondopaminergic human cortical neurons. Dopamine-dependent neurotoxicity is mediated by 54- to 83-kD soluble protein complexes that contain α-synuclein and 14-3-3 protein, which are elevated selectively in the substantia nigra in PD.

Thus, accumulation of soluble α-synuclein protein complexes can render endogenous dopamine toxic, suggesting a potential mechanism for the selectivity of neuronal loss in PD. Inflammatory mechanisms may also play a role, especially in the context of activated microglial cells. Patients with PD have selective degeneration of neurons in the SNc accompanied by microglial activation and a challenged immune system.[10]

Mitochondrial dysfunction and oxidative stress

Mitochondrial dysfunction has been implicated in the pathophysiology of PD. A reduction in mitochondrial complex I activity of 20% to 40% in the SNc has been observed in PD but not in multiple system atrophy.[11] In the rotenone model, there is selective vulnerability of the dopaminergic nigral neurons, possibly related to energetically compromised mitochondria.[12] The neurotoxin N-methyl-4-phenyl-1,2,3,6-tetrahydropyridine (MPTP) also exerts its effect through mitochondrial complex I accumulation. Animal models of PD using MPTP, rotenone, and paraquat have been useful in studying these mechanisms. More recently, a reverse genetic approach with mitochondrial transcription factor A (Tfam) knockout mice has also been used to study this question.[13]

MPTP

The discovery of parkinsonism in addicts following exposure to MPTP led to the MPTP model of PD in various species. The MPTP-lesioned marmoset model in particular has been valuable for the study of PD and response to treatment.[14] The most significant and consistent neurochemical changes occur within the dopamine system. Surviving nigral neurons show reductions in the immunoreactivity of tyrosine hydroxylase with prominent axonal pathology in the nigrostriatal pathway. A striking reduction in dopamine is noted in the striatum and the substantia nigra in MPTP-lesioned monkeys, with lesser levels of depletion seen in the nucleus accumbens and olfactory tubercle. Dopamine depletion has also been reported in the hypothalamus, frontal cortex, and ventral tegmentum.[15] On pathological examination, the cells of the centrolateral area of the SNc are most affected, a state that resembles findings in autopsy studies of PD. The mechanisms by which MPTP induces cell death are manifold.[16] MPTP is rapidly converted in brain cells to its toxic form of MPP+ and undergoes uptake into the mitochondria. Here it blocks the electron transport chain, setting off an early energy crisis followed by a long-term increase in oxidative stress due to increased production of reactive oxidative species, especially superoxide radicals. These react with nitric oxide to produce peroxynitrite, a highly reactive species that damages proteins by oxidation and nitration. Nuclear DNA can also be damaged, with poly- (ADP-ribose) polymerase (PARP) activation playing an important role. It is worth noting that the actual death of SNc neurons is a later process, which suggests that early mechanisms have an indirect effect, provoking activation of apoptotic mechanisms.[17] Based on these strong parallels with PD, the MPTP model has proven to be especially useful in the understanding of etiological factors leading to PD.

Rotenone

Rotenone ("from the roots"), named for its derivation from the roots of the *Lonchocarpus* plant, is used as an organic insecticide. It has a strong inhibitory effect on complex I of the mitochondrial transport chain, thereby inhibiting oxidative phosphorylation. Rotenone infusion into rodents can result in the degeneration of nigrostriatal neurons and the formation of α-synuclein-rich inclusions resembling Lewy bodies. However, rotenone has a short half-life and does not readily leach from soil. Thus it is unlikely to have a direct causal effect in PD, despite its usefulness in animal models.[18]

Paraquat

Paraquat is a widely used herbicide with a chemical structure remarkably similar to MPTP (Fig. 5.2). It is a relatively weak inhibitor of complex I activity compared to rotenone and MPTP. However, it has been shown to increase α-synuclein fibril formation for in vivo models[19] and has been implicated in epidemiological studies as a risk factor for PD.[20] When mice deficient in the DJ-1 gene are treated with paraquat, dopamine loss and motor dysfunction are observed that may be related to decreased proteasome activities and increased ubiquitinated protein levels. These processes were not observed in normal mice treated with paraquat, suggesting a mechanism whereby environmental and genetic factors might interact through proteasome impairment in PD brains, and arguing for a multiple-hit hypothesis of PD.

Tfam knockout mice

Midbrain dopaminergic neurons of PD patients contain high levels of somatic mtDNA mutations, which may impact respiratory chain function. Conditional knockout mice with disruption of the gene for Tfam in dopaminergic neurons have similar reduction in mtDNA expression and respiratory chain deficiency in midbrain dopaminergic neurons.[13] They show a parkinsonian phenotype with adult onset of gradual impairment of motor function with formation of intraneuronal inclusions and death of dopaminergic neurons. These studies further support the importance of mitochondrial respiratory chain dysfunction in PD.

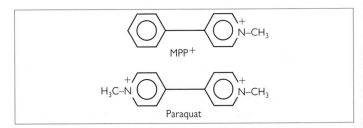

Figure 5.2 Comparison of chemical structures of Paraquat and MPTP.

Environmental factors

Rural living and pesticides

Living in a rural area is believed to increase the incidence of PD, in particular young-onset PD.[21,22] However, not all studies support this association.[23] Working in the agricultural industry is associated with a higher incidence of PD, possibly due to exposure to pesticides and herbicides. In the American Cancer Society's Cancer Prevention Study II Nutrition Cohort, a longitudinal study, individuals who were exposed to pesticides had a 70% higher incidence of PD than those not exposed.[24] The relative risk for pesticide exposure was similar in farmers and nonfarmers. No relationship was found between risk for PD and exposure to asbestos, chemical/acids/solvents, coal or stone dust, or eight other occupational exposures. Among the pesticides and herbicides observed to be potential risk factors are the organochloride dieldrin, dithiocarbamates, rotenone, and paraquat. However, the significant association of farming with PD cannot be explained fully on the basis of pesticide exposure. Other factors such as consumption of well water may further contribute to this association.

Occupational and toxic exposures

Although welding was reported as a risk factor for PD in a case-control study,[25] this has failed to stand up to the scrutiny of well-controlled population-based studies. The Rochester Epidemiology Project found physicians and subjects with nine or more years of education were at significantly increased risk of PD. In contrast, four occupational groups showed a significantly decreased risk of PD: construction and extractive workers (e.g., miners, oil well drillers), production workers (e.g., machine operators, fabricators), metal workers, and engineers.[26] Carbon monoxide poisoning is associated with development of parkinsonism. However, carbon monoxide poisoning is not associated with the aberrant nigrostriatal pathophysiology and Lewy body formation that is the hallmark of idiopathic PD.[27]

While not strictly associated with idiopathic PD, the presence of population clusters associated with parkinsonian phenotypes provides insight into possible etiologies. Atypical parkinsonism in Guadeloupe has been linked to the consumption of fruit and beverages prepared from leaves of *Annona muricata*. Annonacins are lipophilic inhibitors of complex I of the mitochondrial respiratory chain,[28] the toxicity of which includes cell loss of dopaminergic neurons in the SNc.

Infectious etiologies

From 1916 to 1927, an epidemic of an influenza-like illness ravaged Europe and North America. Mortality was up to 40% in those affected, and most survivors developed parkinsonism over the next 10 years.[29] The specific agent causing this pandemic of encephalitis lethargica was never isolated. However, it drew attention to an infectious etiology as a contributor to PD. Interestingly, the possibility that an encephalitis lethargica syndrome is still prevalent has been raised. The suggested mechanism for this syndrome is autoimmunity against deep gray matter neurons.[30]

Some strains of influenza virus A are selectively tropic to the nigral neurons and have been shown to gain access to the brain via nasal passages in mice. Amantadine, an antiviral drug, has been used in managing early PD. In de novo PD patients, amantadine improves peripheral T-cell deficits and cytokine production to normal levels over a 3-month period as well as improving the motor symptoms of PD. Patients with PD who are treated with this drug are reported to exhibit prolonged survival,[31] suggesting a possible neuroprotective effect related to immunomodulation.

Antibodies to the Epstein-Barr virus have shown cross-reactivity with α-synuclein in the brains of patients with PD.[32] Although no evidence of ongoing viral infection in PD has been reported, immunohistochemistry shows reactive microglia, and activated complement components that suggest chronic inflammation occur in affected brain regions in PD.[33] The viral hypothesis has also been invoked to explain the observation of the higher incidence of PD in teachers, medical workers, loggers, and miners.[34] In monozygotic twins discordant for PD, a significantly increased risk was noted in the twins working as teachers or health-care workers.[35] This finding favors an infectious or other environmental etiology, as genetic confounding factors are eliminated. In contrast to these data, the search for viral particles and virus-specific products in the brains of PD patients was not supportive of this hypothesis.[36] Intrauterine exposure to the influenza virus pandemic from 1890 to 1930 was not associated with a subsequent increase in the incidence of PD.[37]

Genetics and gene–environment interactions

The need for genomic investigation in PD is primarily related to the following two facts: (1) a first-degree relative of an affected individual is approximately twice as likely to develop PD versus controls; and (2) the concordance rates in mono- and dizygotic twins are equal in late-onset PD, but much higher in mono- ($\approx$100%) than in dizygotic twins ($\approx$17%) in early-onset PD, which is consistent with early-onset PD having a strong genetic determinant.[35] Thus, there have been two main methods of genomic study. First, families with apparent Mendelian inheritance of PD were investigated using linkage analysis and positional cloning, and five genes have been definitively identified in relation to familial PD. To identify more candidate genes, genomic screens of affected sibling pair families were also undertaken, but these have not produced definitive results. The second method, involving genomic analysis of large populations of sporadic PD patients using single nucleotide polymorphisms, has not resulted in definitive, reproducible PD-related genes. The difficulty in identifying genes using these methods probably relates to the large linkage regions involved, current insufficient genomic coverage, and the genetic heterogeneity of populations with PD (even within families). This last point is consistent with concepts about the involvement of genetics in the pathogenesis of PD in which genetic variability sets the risk of the initiation of the disease process of PD, but a "second hit" involving other factors (e.g., epigenetic phenomena, environmental insults) allows for disease propagation.[6]

Mendelian inheritance of PD

Seven genes have been linked with familial PD (Table 5.1). Five—α-synuclein, parkin, *PINK1*, *DJ-1*, *LRRK2*—have been linked definitively, and the association of the two others—*UCH-L1* and *HTRA2/OMI*—with PD is less well established.

α-synuclein

Three mutations of α-synuclein as well as duplication and triplication of the gene region have been described in familial PD, and genetic variability of the promoter is associated with sporadic PD. Autosomal dominant inheritance of familial PD is observed with mutations of α-synuclein that are consistent with a likely gain of function. The clinical course of affected individuals is similar to sporadic PD, but with an earlier mean age of onset, higher rate of dementia, and some neuropathologic features not common in sporadic PD.[7] The physiologic role of α-synuclein is unclear, but it may be involved in synaptic vesicle recycling, particularly involving dopamine storage. The pathological role of α-synuclein in PD is also not known, but α-synuclein is a major component of Lewy bodies observed in postmortem studies of the brains of individuals with PD.[6]

Parkin

The parkin gene is the second largest gene known, and a wide variety of mutations have been found in familial PD.[38] Parkin is mutated in ≈50% of autosomal-recessive early-onset PD and in ≈70% of sporadic PD with onset less than 20 years, which is consistent with a likely loss of function. The clinical course of affected individuals is typically characterized by early onset, slow progression, and good response to dopaminergic therapy.[38,39] There is, however, a wide variability in the age of onset within some families, indicating the possible importance of epigenetic and environmental factors in influencing the phenotype associated with a given mutation. The physiological role of parkin is thought to relate to its function as a ubiquitin ligase that is important in normal cellular protein degradation pathways.[6] Deficiency in this function may underlie the pathology associated with mutant parkin, including possible disruption of microtubule and mitochondrial function, proteasomal degradation, and neuroprotection with some evidence to suggest susceptibility specific to dopaminergic neurons.

PINK1

Mutations of *PINK1* are centered primarily in and near to the putative kinase domain, and are thought to result in loss of kinase function consistent with the observed autosomal-recessive inheritance pattern.[39] The clinical course in affected individuals typically demonstrates disease onset at <50 years with what are otherwise mostly classical features of sporadic PD. The physiological role of *PINK1* is thought to involve regulation of the electron transport chain and maintenance of mitochondrial membrane potential, particularly as it pertains to the apoptotic signaling cascade. The

Table 5.1 Genetic forms of Parkinson's disease

Locus	Chromosome	Gene product	Inheritance	Age of onset (y)	Clinical features	Pathological features
PARK1 and PARK4	4q21–q23	α-synuclein	AD	Range, 30 to 60; mean, 45	Levodopa-responsive; rapid progression; comorbid dementia	Neuronal loss in SNc and locus ceruleus; Lewy bodies range from few to extensive in triplication cases
PARK2	6q25.2–q27	Parkin	Usually AR	Range, 7 to 58; mean, 26	Levodopa-respession; slow progression; severe dyskinesias; foot dystonia	Neuronal loss in SNc and locus ceruleus; usually Lewy-body negative
PARK5	4p14	Ubiquitin C-terminal hydrolase L1	AD	49 to 50	Typical PD	Lewy bodies reported in a single case
PARK6	1p35–1p36	PINK1	AR	Range, 32 to 48	Levodopa-responsive; slow progression	Undetermined
PARK7	1p36	DJ-1	AR	Range, 20 to 40s; mean, mid-30s	Levodopa-responsive; slow progression; psychiatric symptoms	Undetermined
PARK8	12p11.2–12q31.1	Dardarin/LRRK2	AD	Range, 35 to 79; mean, 57	Typical PD; dementia; features of motor neuron disease	SNc neurodegeneration; with or without Lewy bodies; tau inclusions and neurofibrillary tangles may be seen

AD, autosomal dominant; AR, autosomal recessive; SNc, substantia nigra pars compacta. *Source:* Olanow CW, McNaught KS. Ubiquitin-proteasome system and Parkinson's disease. *Mov Disord.* 2006;21(11):1806–1823.

pathology that results from mutations of *PINK1* may relate to mitochondrial dysfunction in response to oxidative stress, possibly involving parkin.[38]

DJ-1

Multiple types of mutations of *DJ-1* have been found, and inheritance is autosomal-recessive.[39] Affected individuals typically have age of onset around 20 to 40 years, with mostly classical parkinsonian symptoms. They usually respond to dopaminergic therapy. *DJ-1* is thought to play a role as an antioxidant and sensor of oxidative stress, but it may also be involved in protein degradation pathways and apoptotic signaling, possibly in conjunction with parkin and *PINK1*. Furthermore, dysfunction of *DJ-1* may affect these pathways in a manner that preferentially involves dopaminergic neurons.[38]

LRRK2

Mutations are found throughout *LRRK2*'s functional domains. The most common mutant is relatively frequent in both familial autosomal-dominant PD (≈5%) and sporadic PD (≈1.5%). *LRRK2* mutations result in parkinsonism that is very similar to classical PD, and penetrance of symptoms is very tightly linked with aging, which is also similar to idiopathic PD.[38] The physiologic role of *LRRK2* is thought to involve its putative kinase and GTPase activity. Mutant forms have shown increased kinase activity consistent with a gain of function that is often seen in autosomal dominant diseases. Despite the relatively uniform classic parkinsonism seen with *LRRK2* mutations, the neuropathology is quite diverse, which suggests that *LRRK2* dysfunction may be important in the initiation of altered function of multiple cellular systems with a final common pathway resulting in dopaminergic cell death.[6]

UCH-L1 and HTRA2/OMI

It is unclear whether a mutation of *UCH-L1* that has been identified in several families is truly involved in PD.[6] This is due to the failure of the mutation to segregate with disease in one family and the failure of other mutations to be identified despite extensive screening. It is intriguing, however, that a polymorphism in this gene may protect against development of PD, possibly through alteration of interaction of *UCH-L1* with α-synuclein. *HTRA2/OMI* mutations were found in several patients with sporadic PD, and polymorphisms in this gene are found more frequently in patients with PD. However, mutations of *HTRA2/OMI* are not found in families with mutations in the same genetic locus, and so its involvement in PD is not definitively established.

Susceptibility genes

In addition to causative genes, there is recent interest in the role of susceptibility genes. The β-glucocerebrosidase (GBA) gene was found to be a susceptibility gene for PD. About 14% of PD patients were found to carry GBA mutations, compared with 5% of controls. Mutations were found in 22% of PD patients with onset before the age of 50 years and in 10% of those with later onset.[40] The *LRRK2* Gly2385Arg mutation may be a risk factor for PD in the Chinese population.[41] The clinical impact of these and similar findings remains to be defined.

Genetic testing in PD

Commercially available genetic testing for familial PD is available for certain sequence variations in the parkin, *PINK1*, and *LRRK2* genes. Genetic testing for PD is largely uninformative, as many affected individuals will not possess these specific mutations. Therefore, negative testing does not exclude familial PD. Routine genetic testing is not recommended. Genetic testing may be of value in young-onset PD where parkin mutations may account for ≈80% in those under 20 years and ≈25% in those aged 20 to 30. Autosomal PD due to the *LRRK2* mutation may be demonstrated in 18% to 30% of those of Ashkenazi Jewish and North African Arab backgrounds.[42]

References

1. Parkinson J. *An Essay on the Shaking Palsy.* London: Sherwood, Neeley and Jones; 1817.

2. Gower W. *A Manual of Diseases of the Nervous System.* Philadelphia, PA: P Blakiston; 1888.

3. Tanner CM, Ottman R, Goldman SM, et al. Parkinson disease in twins: an etiologic study. *JAMA.* 1999;281(4):341–346.

4. Polymeropoulos MH, Lavedan C, Leroy E, et al. Mutation in the alpha-synuclein gene identified in families with Parkinson's disease. *Science.* 1997;276(5321):2045–2047.

5. Wang HQ, Takahashi R. Expanding insights on the involvement of endoplasmic reticulum stress in Parkinson's disease. *Antioxid Redox Signal.* 2007;9(5):553–561.

6. Moore DJ, West AB, Dawson VL, Dawson TM. Molecular pathophysiology of Parkinson's disease. *Annu Rev Neurosci.* 2005;28:57–87.

7. Olanow CW, McNaught KS. Ubiquitin-proteasome system and Parkinson's disease. *Mov Disord.* 2006;21(11):1806–1823.

8. Hebert SS, De Strooper B. Molecular biology. miRNAs in neurodegeneration. *Science.* 2007;317(5842):1179–1180.

9. Cuervo AM, Stefanis L, Fredenburg R, Lansbury PT, Sulzer D. Impaired degradation of mutant alpha-synuclein by chaperone-mediated autophagy. *Science.* 2004;305(5688):1292–1295.

10. Orr CF, Rowe DB, Halliday GM. An inflammatory review of Parkinson's disease. *Prog Neurobiol.* 2002;68(5):325–340.

11. Schapira AH, Mann VM, Cooper JM, et al. Anatomic and disease specificity of NADH CoQ1 reductase (complex I) deficiency in Parkinson's disease. *J Neurochem.* 1990;55(6):2142–2145.

12. Kristal BS, Conway AD, Brown AM, et al. Selective dopaminergic vulnerability: 3,4-dihydroxyphenylacetaldehyde targets mitochondria. *Free Radic Biol Med.* 2001;30(8):924–931.

13. Ekstrand MI, Terzioglu M, Galter D, et al. Progressive parkinsonism in mice with respiratory-chain-deficient dopamine neurons. *Proc Natl Acad Sci USA.* 2007;104(4):1325–1330.

14. Langston JW, Langston EB, Irwin I. MPTP-induced parkinsonism in human and non-human primates—clinical and experimental aspects. *Acta Neurol Scand.* 1984;100(suppl):49–54.

15. Gibb WR, Lees AJ, Jenner P, Marsden CD. The dopamine neurotoxin 1-methyl-4-phenyl-1,2,3,6-tetrahydropyridine (MPTP) produces histological lesions in the hypothalamus of the common marmoset. *Neurosci Lett.* 1986;65(1):79–83.

16. Dauer W, Przedborski S. Parkinson's disease: mechanisms and models. *Neuron.* 2003;39(6):889–909.

17. Jackson-Lewis V, Jakowec M, Burke RE, Przedborski S. Time course and morphology of dopaminergic neuronal death caused by the neurotoxin 1-methyl-4-phenyl-1,2,3,6-tetrahydropyridine. *Neurodegeneration.* 1995;4(3):257–269.

18. Bove J, Prou D, Perier C, Przedborski S. Toxin-induced models of Parkinson's disease. *NeuroRx.* 2005;2(3):484–494.

19. Manning-Bog AB, McCormack AL, Li J, Uversky VN, Fink AL, Di Monte DA. The herbicide paraquat causes up-regulation and aggregation of alpha-synuclein in mice: paraquat and alpha-synuclein. *J Biol Chem.* 2002;277(3):1641–1644.

20. Liou HH, Tsai MC, Chen CJ, et al. Environmental risk factors and Parkinson's disease: a case-control study in Taiwan. *Neurology.* 1997;48(6):1583–1588.

21. Rajput AH, Uitti RJ, Stern W, et al. Geography, drinking water chemistry, pesticides and herbicides and the etiology of Parkinson's disease. *Can J Neurol Sci.* 1987;14(3 Suppl):414–418.

22. Behari M, Srivastava AK, Das RR, Pandey RM. Risk factors of Parkinson's disease in Indian patients. *J Neurol Sci.* 2001;190(1/2):49–55.

23. Semchuk KM, Love EJ, Lee RG. Parkinson's disease and exposure to rural environmental factors: a population based case-control study. *Can J Neurol Sci.* 1991;18(3):279–286.

24. Ascherio A, Chen H, Weisskopf MG, et al. Pesticide exposure and risk for Parkinson's disease. *Ann Neurol.* 2006;60(2):197–203.

25. Racette BA, McGee-Minnich L, Moerlein SM, Mink JW, Videen TO, Perlmutter JS. Welding-related parkinsonism: clinical features, treatment, and pathophysiology. *Neurology.* 2001;56(1):8–13.

26. Frigerio R, Elbaz A, Sanft KR, et al. Education and occupations preceding Parkinson disease: a population-based case-control study. *Neurology.* 2005;65(10):1575–83.

27. Choi IS. Parkinsonism after carbon monoxide poisoning. *Eur Neurol.* 2002;48(1):30–33.

28. Champy P, Hoglinger GU, Feger J, et al. Annonacin, a lipophilic inhibitor of mitochondrial complex I, induces nigral and striatal neurodegeneration in rats: possible relevance for atypical parkinsonism in Guadeloupe. *J Neurochem.* 2004;88(1):63–69.

29. Ransmayr G. Constantin von Economo's contribution to the understanding of movement disorders. *Mov Disord.* 2007;22(4):469–475.

30. Yamada T, Yamanaka I, Nakajima S. Immunohistochemistry of a cytoplasmic dynein (MAP 1C)-like molecule in rodent and human brain tissue: an example of molecular mimicry between cytoplasmic dynein and influenza A virus. *Acta Neuropathol (Berl).* 1996;92(3):306–311.

31. Uitti RJ, Rajput AH, Ahlskog JE, et al. Amantadine treatment is an independent predictor of improved survival in Parkinson's disease. *Neurology.* 1996;46(6):1551–1556.

32. Woulfe J, Hoogendoorn H, Tarnopolsky M, Munoz DG. Monoclonal antibodies against Epstein-Barr virus cross-react with alpha-synuclein in human brain. *Neurology.* 2000;55(9):1398–1401.

33. McGeer PL, Yasojima K, McGeer EG. Inflammation in Parkinson's disease. *Adv Neurol.* 2001;86:83–89.

34. Kumar A, Calne SM, Schulzer M, et al. Clustering of Parkinson disease: shared cause or coincidence? *Arch Neurol.* 2004;61(7):1057–1060.

35. Tanner CM. Is the cause of Parkinson's disease environmental or hereditary? Evidence from twin studies. *Adv Neurol.* 2003;91:133–142.

36. Schwartz J, Elizan TS. Search for viral particles and virus-specific products in idiopathic Parkinson disease brain material. *Ann Neurol.* 1979;6(3):261–263.

37. Ebmeier KP, Mutch WJ, Calder SA, Crawford JR, Stewart L, Besson JO. Does idiopathic parkinsonism in Aberdeen follow intrauterine influenza? *J Neurol Neurosurg Psychiatry.* 1989;52(7):911–913.

38. Gosal D, Ross OA, Toft M. Parkinson's disease: the genetics of a heterogeneous disorder. *Eur J Neurol.* 2006;13(6):616–627.

39. Kubo S, Hattori N, Mizuno Y. Recessive Parkinson's disease. *Mov Disord.* 2006;21(7):885–893.

40. Clark LN, Ross BM, Wang Y, et al. Mutations in the glucocerebrosidase gene are associated with early-onset Parkinson disease. *Neurology.* 2007; 69(12):1270–1277.

41. Skipper L, Li Y, Bonnard C, et al. Comprehensive evaluation of common genetic variation within LRRK2 reveals evidence for association with sporadic Parkinson's disease. *Hum Mol Genet.* 2005;14(23):3549–3556.

42. Lorincz MT. Clinical implications of Parkinson's disease genetics. *Semin Neurol.* 2006;26(5):492–498.

Chapter 6

Approach to the treatment of early Parkinson's disease

Stewart Isaacson

The choice of initial therapy for treating early Parkinson's disease is best individualized after consultation with the patient, family members, and other caregivers. Patients can report how they feel and how motor and nonmotor symptoms affect their experiences of daily life. Their families and caregivers can relate observations of symptoms of which the patient may not be aware, such as rest tremor or confusion.

Integration of nonpharmacological and wellness strategies should be a focus from the outset.[1] Incorporation of regular exercise into daily activities must be a priority. Regular courses of rehabilitative therapies may be useful. Proper nutrition, stress management, and coping techniques should be emphasized throughout the course of any chronic disorder.

Often, pharmacological therapy does not need to be initiated during the time in which a patient awaits neurological consultation, ancillary assessments, or a confirmatory opinion. Even upon clear diagnosis, some patients and their physicians choose to delay beginning dopaminergic medication. The reasons for this may include fear of adverse effects, polypharmacy, insignificant symptoms, and the stigma of requiring daily medication. However, fears about toxicity of some of the medications (such as levodopa) that are used to treat Parkinson's disease have generally been proved unfounded and should no longer be allowed to delay institution of appropriate treatment.[2] To date, no convincing laboratory or clinical evidence of levodopa toxicity has emerged, and some evidence may even suggest that levodopa is neuroprotective.

Pharmacological agents used in the treatment of early PD

In addition to carbidopa/levodopa (CD/LD), many medication options exist to treat early PD, including several newer medications (Table 6.1). Options include anticholinergics, amantadine, selective monoamine oxidase type B (MAO-B) inhibitors, dopamine agonists, CD/LD with catechol-O-methyl transferase (COMT) inhibitor, and potential neuroprotective agents.[1]

Table 6.1 Common medications useful for treating early Parkinson's disease
Levodopa-containing medication
Carbidopa/levodopa (Sinemet IR, Parcopa)
Sustained-release carbidopa/levodopa (Sinemet CR)
Carbidopa/levodopa/entacapone (Stalevo)
Dopamine agonists
Pramipexole (Mirapex)
Ropinirole (Requip)
Ropinirole XL (Requip XL)
MAO-B inhibitors
Rasagiline (Azilect)
Selegiline (Eldepryl)
Amantadine

Anticholinergics

Anticholinergics, such as trihexyphenidyl (Artane), typically have modest effects on symptom control.[1] Their effect on tremor may sometimes be more robust, especially in patients with younger onset, tremor-predominant disease. Unfortunately, increasing dosages are associated with limiting, adverse effects of dry mouth, constipation, somnolence, and memory impairment. This class of medications is therefore rarely used. The usual starting dose for trihexyphenidyl is 2 mg tid, and the dose is increased as tolerated up to approximately 15 mg/day.

Amantadine

Amantadine (Symmetrel) has a mild antiparkinsonian effect, especially on tremor.[1] Its mechanism of action is unclear, and may involve both anticholinergic and glutamatergic effects. It is typically well tolerated when used at a dose of 100 mg at breakfast and lunch, but older patients may have a higher incidence of adverse effects with the twice-daily dosing, including constipation, confusion, and hallucinations. Amantadine has mainly renal clearance, and reduced creatine clearance with aging may increase adverse effects.

Monoamine oxidase type B (MAO-B) inhibitors

Selective MAO-B inhibitors reduce the breakdown of dopamine in the brain, thus enhancing levels of endogenous dopamine being produced by surviving dopaminergic neurons.[3] There are presently three selective MAO-B inhibitors available: selegiline (Eldepryl), rasagiline (Azilect), and buccal-absorbed orally disintegrating selegiline (Zelapar). There are no data regarding the use of orally disintegrating selegiline in early disease. This class of medications usually provides only modest benefit in many patients. Adverse effects are uncommon when MAO-B inhibitors are used as monotherapy but can include orthostatic hypotension, nausea, and fatigue. Selegiline may also cause insomnia, perhaps related to amphetamine metabolites.

The MAO-B inhibitor selegiline was one of the first medications used to study neuroprotection in PD. The Deprenyl and Tocopherol Antioxidative Therapy for PD (DATATOP) study compared initial therapy with selegiline to placebo.[3] A modest symptomatic effect lasting 6 to 9 months confounded assessment of potential neuroprotective property. More recently, a prospective study using the delayed-start design was performed with the MAO-B inhibitor rasagiline.[4] In this study, the group that initially received placebo followed by an active drug after a 6-month delay did not achieve the full benefit of the earlier initiated group. This may suggest a neuroprotective effect. Studies using the delayed-start design are ongoing with rasagiline to confirm this result.

One of the major limitations regarding the use of MAO-B inhibitors is that certain medications, such as meperidine, tramadol, methadone, propoxyphene, cold medications, and weight-reducing medications that contain vasoconstrictors, are contraindicated with their use. The usual dose for selegiline is 5 mg with breakfast and lunch. The standard dose of rasagiline is 1 mg once a day.

Dopamine agonists

Dopamine agonists directly stimulate the postsynaptic dopamine receptors. Extensive work has been done to investigate the role of dopamine agonists as monotherapy in the treatment of early PD.[5] Initially, these drugs were developed as adjunctive therapy to levodopa to provide more consistent benefit with fewer adverse effects. Later, they were used to delay initiation of levodopa and motor complications. Studies have provided evidence that the initial use of dopamine agonists prior to beginning levodopa is associated with reduced emergence of motor complications.[6] Whether this is due to a reduction in the incidence of motor complications or to a delay in their emergence remains unclear. Both dyskinesia and end-of-dose "wearing off" are reduced with the administration of dopamine agonists. This apparent benefit of using a dopamine agonist before beginning levodopa appears to persist through the first 10 years of therapy, but long-term follow-up is not robust, and the later introduction of levodopa may hasten the emergence of both symptoms.

Adverse effects of oral dopamine agonists may be idiosyncratic, occur at peak drug level (C_{max}), or reflect accumulation effects. In contrast to idiosyncratic reactions, peak adverse effects are predictable, occurring 1.5 to 2 hours after a dose. These occur mainly during titration and are minimized by slowing dose escalation to allow for the development of tolerance. Tolerance may develop within 4 to 5 days, but the adverse effects may reappear as the dosage is titrated upward. Adverse events for agonists include nausea, vomiting, dizziness, somnolence, insomnia, pedal edema, orthostatic hypotension, hallucinations, confusion, mood changes, euphoria, vivid dreams, and sleep problems. There have also been reports of unexpected sleep episodes and impulsive behaviors such as gambling, shopping, sexual behaviors and eating. Some of these adverse effects may be lessened by administering the medication with a meal. Although the oral dopamine agonists are used three times a day, using them twice daily (morning and bedtime) can reduce the number of peak dose adverse events that occur during waking hours. The newer transdermal dopamine agonist rotigotine (Neupro) delivers a stable plasma level over 24 hours without a peak concentration, so it may cause fewer peak dose–related adverse effects. Rotigotine has been withdrawn from the U.S. market due to crystallization of the drug on the patch.

The early oral dopamine agonists bromocriptine (Parlodel) and pergolide (Permax) were ergot-derived, with risk of ergot-induced fibrosis, including cardiac valvular fibrosis. Pergolide has been withdrawn from the U.S. market, and bromocriptine is rarely used due to this potential risk. The newer dopamine agonists pramipexole (Mirapex) and ropinirole (Requip) are nonergoline compounds, and presumably devoid of this potential risk. Pramipexole is initiated at 0.125 mg 3 times per day and is increased over 7 weeks to a maximum dose of 1.5 mg 3 times per day. Ropinirole is initiated at 0.25 mg 3 times per day and is gradually increased over 12 weeks to a maximum dose of 8 mg 3 times per day. Ropinirole XL (Requip XL), a once-a-day preparation of ropinirole, was recently approved for treatment of PD. Ropinirole XL is started at 2 mg once a day and is increased by 2 mg every 1 to 2 weeks, to a maximum of 24 mg per day.

Levodopa

After 40 years of use in PD, levodopa remains a viable option for treating early PD.[1] When combined with the peripheral decarboxylase inhibitor carbidopa (Lodosyn), the robust clinical effects, relatively low cost, and reasonable tolerability profile of levodopa support its early use. The combination of CD/LD with the COMT inhibitor entacapone (Comtan, or in a combination pill with CD/LD as Stalevo) is being compared to CD/LD alone in a multicenter study to assess the emergence of motor complications. The rationale behind combining COMT inhibitors and CD/LD is that the inhibitors are thought to improve the availability of levodopa in the body and extend the duration of action of each levodopa dose, thereby increasing the amount of time over which the symptoms of PD are well controlled.

Despite rarely being of clinical relevance in early PD, timing of levodopa administration and meals is frequently discussed. Levodopa absorption in the intestinal tract may be reduced if the medication is taken together with protein, but this effect is more important in advancing disease. Gastroparesis may cause a delayed levodopa effect, but clinical symptoms are not usually apparent from this in early PD. Distinct from later PD, the timing of levodopa doses in early PD often does not result in motor fluctuations or wearing off.

Initiation of treatment should be approached with the goal of maximizing clinical efficacy of the selected medication while minimizing potential adverse effects. Patients can gain confidence through the slow introduction of the medication. Patients should be reassured that tolerance to dopaminergic adverse effects usually develops rapidly. Robust improvement may be seen in days or weeks after beginning levodopa, but it may take several weeks or longer with dopamine agonists. It is important to manage expectations of the patient and caregivers so that medications are not stopped before benefits begin and adverse effects wane.

Carbidopa/levodopa is available in 10/100, 25/100, and 25/250 mg doses and in sustained-release preparations of 25/100 and 50/200 mg, where the first number is the milligram dose of carbidopa and the second number is the amount of levodopa. Carbidopa/levodopa is usually initiated at half of a 25/100 mg tablet twice a day and initially increased to one tablet 3 times a day. The dose is gradually increased as needed. Once treatment has led to significant symptom improvement, the dose can be maintained. If improvement is suboptimal, the dose should be slowly increased. The goal of instituting treatment should be to improve symptoms to as close to normal as possible, without causing intolerable adverse effects. This is not always possible: sensitivity to dopaminergic medication, idiosyncratic reactions, suboptimal improvement, and patient noncompliance may hinder effective treatment strategies in the early stages of PD.

One of the major limitations of the long-term use of levodopa is the development of motor fluctuations and dyskinesia.[7] These motor complications occur in approximately 50% of PD patients after 5 years of levodopa use. When levodopa is initiated, the PD symptoms are generally controlled during the day. Eventually, however, usually over a period of months, ingestion of a levodopa dose improves the PD symptoms for only a few hours, and then the PD symptoms reemerge. This is known as end-of-dose wearing-off. As the disease progresses, the benefit with each dose of levodopa decreases. In addition, patients develop random on/off fluctuations. These are rapid transitions (over seconds) between the "on state" and "off state." Levodopa therapy can also lead to dyskinesias, which are involuntary movements such as chorea, dystonia, and ballismus. Other common, acute adverse effects with carbidopa/levodopa include nausea, vomiting, somnolence, hallucination, and orthostatic hypotension. Rare side effects include skin rash, diaphoresis, cardiac arrhythmias, and pedal edema.

Decision tree for the choice of PD treatment

Some believe that delaying dopaminergic therapy may not be beneficial. Appropriate pharmacotherapy improves motor and nonmotor symptoms, allowing patients to maintain optimal functioning in daily activities and enhancing quality of life. Attempts to identify biomarkers may allow therapies to begin prior to the emergence of clear motor symptoms, and such biomarkers would be particularly important if a potent neuroprotectant could be identified. However, at the present time treatment is based on improving symptoms rather than slowing the disease course.

Despite a lack of prospective controlled studies, consensus is growing to support earlier initiation of treatment, ideally beginning the selected treatment as soon as a patient would benefit from it. Ongoing work suggests that the onset of clinical (motor) parkinsonism is preceded by more widespread neuropathological changes and by nonmotor symptoms, so there may be more to gain from treatment than just motor improvement.

Recent algorithms have emerged that form a consensus on initial therapy for PD (Fig. 6.1). Nonpharmacological therapies are important to

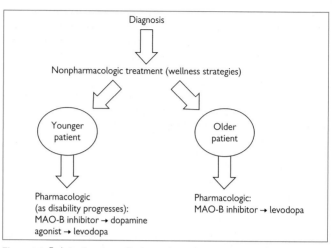

Figure 6.1 Early treatment paradigm.

incorporate early in the treatment plan. Daily exercise may help optimize mobility, flexibility, and stability. Good nutrition and stress management will augment coping strategies needed to help deal with having a chronic, progressive neurological disorder. A multidisciplinary team approach can be used to coordinate wellness strategies.

At some point, pharmacological treatment is initiated. The timing of this is based on an assessment of how symptoms affect the patient's functional activities of daily life, employment, and quality of life. Once the decision to begin symptomatic treatment is made, delaying medication or using suboptimal dosages is not warranted. Usually when patients have mild symptoms that are not causing significant functional impairment, it is reasonable to initiate therapy with MAO-B inhibitors. Although MAO-B inhibitors have mild symptomatic benefits, they are also well tolerated as monotherapy.

Once there is significant functional impairment, the goal of symptomatic treatment is to improve tremor, rigidity, bradykinesia, gait, and mobility without causing intolerable adverse effects. CD/LD may be the most effective medication to accomplish these goals, but a number of studies have suggested that initiating a dopamine agonist prior to beginning CD/LD may be a better strategy in some patients. These studies provide evidence that the emergence of motor complications (dyskinesia and wearing off) may be delayed when dopaminergic therapy in PD is begun with a dopamine agonist instead of CD/LD. However, older patients are more prone to the acute adverse effects with dopamine agonists and hence may be more appropriate candidates for initiating treatment with levodopa.

For now, based on this body of evidence, it has become reasonable to initiate symptomatic dopaminergic therapy with either CD/LD or a dopamine agonist.[8] Emerging consensus supports the early use of a dopamine agonist in younger patients, adding CD/LD if the therapeutic effect is not robust or is limited by the occurrence of adverse effects.

Some patients may not be good candidates for dopamine agonists. For example, low or orthostatic blood pressures may be exacerbated by dopamine agonists. Memory impairment may also be worsened. Daytime somnolence or a history of a sleep disorder such as sleep apnea may predispose the patient to intolerable excessive daytime somnolence with a dopamine agonist. Finally, as mentioned earlier, advancing age should also be considered, as there seems to be a lower incidence of developing dyskinesia when PD onset occurs after the age of 70. The availability of 24-hour transdermal and oral formulations of dopamine agonists may be associated with fewer peak side effects and better overall tolerability, allowing their more widespread use in early PD.

Summary

The treatment of early PD is optimized by careful and persistent attention to nonpharmacological wellness strategies coupled with an individualized approach to pharmacological therapies based on impairment of function, quality, and activities of daily life. The use of selective MAO-B inhibitors can provide mild symptomatic improvement, and may potentially have neuroprotective effects. The addition of a dopamine agonist provides symptomatic benefit and may delay the emergence of motor complications when begun prior to CD/LD. The eventual addition of CD/LD typically provides robust symptomatic benefit.

References

1. Olanow CW, Watts RL, Koller WC. An algorithm (decision tree) for the management of Parkinson's disease: treatment guidelines. *Neurology.* 2001;56(suppl):S1–S88.

2. Parkinson Study Group. Levodopa and the progression of Parkinson's disease. *N Engl J Med.* 2004;351(24):2498–2508.

3. Parkinson Study Group. DATATOP: a multicenter controlled clinical trial in early Parkinson's disease. *Arch Neurol.* 1989;46(10):1052–1060.

4. Parkinson Study Group. A controlled, randomized, delayed-start study of rasagiline in early Parkinson disease. *Arch Neurol.* 2004;61:561–566.

5. Adler CH, Sethi KD, Hauser RA, et al. Ropinirole for the treatment of early Parkinson's disease. The Ropinirole Study Group. *Neurology.* 1997;49(2):393–399.

6. Parkinson Study Group. Pramipexole vs levodopa as initial treatment for Parkinson disease: a randomized controlled trial. *JAMA.* 2000;284(15):1931–1938.

7. Rascol O, Brooks DJ, Korczyn AD, et al. A five-year study of the incidence of dyskinesia in patients with early Parkinson's disease who were treated with ropinirole or levodopa. 056 Study Group. *N Engl J Med.* 2000;342(20):1484–1491.

8. Miyasaki JM, Martin W, Suchowersky O, Weiner WJ, Lang AE. Practice parameter: initiation of treatment for Parkinson's disease: an evidence-based review: report of the Quality Standards Subcommittee of the American Academy of Neurology. *Neurology.* 2002;58(1):11–7.

Chapter 7

Management of motor disability in advanced Parkinson's disease

Kelly E. Lyons and Rajesh Pahwa

Parkinson's disease (PD) is a progressive neurodegenerative disorder with increasing disability as the disease progresses. Motor disability in advanced disease can be related to either complications of antiparkinsonian therapy or to the progression of the disease. Motor complications related to levodopa therapy include motor fluctuations and dyskinesia. Disease progression often results in the development of postural instability and freezing.[1]

Levodopa is currently the most effective treatment for PD and is required by almost all patients as the disease advances. Levodopa is combined with a decarboxylase inhibitor, carbidopa, to increase the amount of levodopa that reaches the brain and to reduce side effects of nausea and vomiting.[1] Carbidopa/levodopa (Sinemet, Parcopa) is available in tablets with strengths of 10/100, 25/100, and 25/250 mg. Extended-release carbidopa/levodopa is available in strengths of 25/100 and 50/200 mg.

Nearly all PD patients have a good, stable response to levodopa for the first few years of therapy. However, prolonged use of levodopa leads to motor complications that can cause significant disability and greatly impact daily functioning and quality of life.[2] One study demonstrated that 40% of patients developed levodopa-induced motor complications after 5 years of therapy, and this increased to 100% after 10 years.[3] Risk factors for the development of levodopa-induced motor complications are younger age of PD onset, greater disease severity, higher daily doses of levodopa, and longer disease duration.[4] Levodopa-induced motor complications include motor fluctuations and dyskinesia (Table 7.1).

Motor fluctuations

Motor fluctuations are alternations between "on" time, when symptoms are well controlled, and "off" time, when the medication is less effective and parkinsonian symptoms return.[1] End-of-dose wearing-off, the most common type of motor fluctuation, is a decrease in the duration of effectiveness of a single levodopa dose. When levodopa is initiated, patients generally experience a stable control of symptoms without deterioration between doses. As PD progresses, symptoms begin to return toward the

Table 7.1 Levodopa-induced motor complications

Motor fluctuations	Alterations between good control of symptoms and poor or no control of symptoms
End-of-dose wearing-off	PD symptoms reemerge toward the end of the previous levodopa dose
On/off phenomenon	Random, sudden periods when PD symptoms occur
Delayed "on"	Extended period of time required for a dose of levodopa to improve PD symptoms
Dose failures	Individual dose of levodopa does not provide usual benefit
Dyskinesia	Involuntary movements, namely choreatic
Peak dose dyskinesia	Involuntary movements occurring at the peak plasma levodopa concentration
Diphasic dyskinesia	Involuntary movements occurring when plasma levodopa levels are rising and falling
Dystonia	Dystonic symptoms

PD, Parkinson's disease.

end of a levodopa dose and do not resolve until the next dose is taken. End-of-dose wearing-off is a gradual and predictable return of symptoms. Over time, it occurs earlier and earlier, so that the duration of the levodopa effect becomes shorter. As PD progresses, off periods become more common, can start suddenly, and are no longer predictably based on the timing of the levodopa dose. This is called the on/off phenomenon. In addition, the time period before a levodopa dose begins to take effect can increase, known as a "delayed on," and in some cases a given dose may have no effect at all; this is known as a dose failure, or "no on." Freezing of gait refers to the feeling that one's feet are stuck to the floor. This is characterized by an inability to move, which can lead to falling. Freezing often occurs when initiating movement, referred to as start hesitation, or when turning or going through doorways, as well as in other small or crowded spaces. Freezing can occur in both the on and off states. Off-state freezing is related to fluctuations in levodopa response; however, on-state freezing does not appear to be the result of levodopa intake or response.

Dyskinesia

Dyskinesia are involuntary, most commonly choreatic, movements that can involve the face, head, neck, arms, legs, torso, and respiratory muscles.[1] The most common type of dyskinesia is peak dose dyskinesia, which occur as levodopa blood levels reach the highest concentration. This type of dyskinesia has been referred to as improvement-dyskinesia-improvement (I-D-I). Less commonly, diphasic dyskinesia occur in which dyskinesia are present at the beginning of the levodopa dose cycle, when the patient is starting to "turn on," and again at the end of the dose cycle as the patient begins to "wear off," but are not present at peak levodopa concentration. This type of dyskinesia has been referred to as dyskinesia-improvement-dyskinesia (D-I-D) and affects approximately 15% to 20% of patients with dyskinesia. Dyskinesia can also present as dystonia, which involves abnormal, uncomfortable posturing, most often of the distal arms or legs. Dystonia most commonly occurs while levodopa plasma levels are either increasing or decreasing and can therefore be seen in both the on and the off states.

Motor complications: Management

The goal of managing advanced PD is to maintain stable control of symptoms while avoiding motor complications. This can be a challenge, as treatment adjustments to reduce off time need to be made without causing an increase in dyskinesia, and attempts to reduce dyskinesia should not increase off time. There are multiple treatment options for PD patients experiencing levodopa-induced motor complications (Tables 7.2 and 7.3). The American Academy of Neurology (AAN),[4] Movement Disorder Society (MDS),[5] and European Federation of Neurological Societies (EFNS)[6] have each published guidelines for the treatment of advanced PD patients with motor complications (Table 7.4). These guidelines are based on the published literature and are largely influenced by the quality and amount of information published for each study, and they may not necessarily reflect the most common clinical practices.

There are multiple treatment options to reduce motor complications, including adjusting levodopa dosing or formulation; addition of a monoamine oxidase type B (MAO-B) inhibitor, dopamine agonist, catechol-O-methyl transferase (COMT) inhibitor, or amantadine; and, when medication changes are not successful, deep brain stimulation (Tables 7.2 and 7.3).

Levodopa

One strategy to reduce motor complications, particularly end-of-dose wearing-off, is to use smaller, more frequent doses of levodopa if dyskinesia are present or higher individual doses if there are no dyskinesia. Levodopa

Table 7.2 Treatment strategies for motor fluctuations and dyskinesia
Motor fluctuations
• Increase dosage or frequency of levodopa
• Switch to extended-release levodopa
• Adjunctive therapies
• MAO-B inhibitors (rasagiline, selegiline, orally disintegrating selegiline)
• Dopamine agonists (pramipexole, ropinirole, apomorphine)
• COMT inhibitors (entacapone, tolcapone)
• Deep brain stimulation
Dyskinesia
• Decrease individual dose of levodopa
• Amantadine
• Deep brain stimulation

COMT, catechol-O-methyl transferase; MAO-B, monoamine oxidase type B.

Table 7.3 Treatment options for levodopa-induced motor complications

Treatment (Refs.)	Available strengths	Titration/dose ranges	Daily "off" time reduction[a]
MAO-B inhibitors			
Rasagiline (Azilect) (7,8)	0.5, 1.0 mg tablets	Start with 0.5 mg qd and increase to 1.0 mg qd if necessary	8% to 14% 0.5 to 1.0 h
Selegiline (Eldepryl)	5 mg capsules	5 mg bid (breakfast and lunch)	Insufficient data
Orally disintegrating selegiline (Zelapar) (9)	1.25 mg dissolvable tablets	Start with 1.25 mg qd and increase to 2.5 mg qd after 6 weeks if necessary	23% 1.6 h
Dopamine agonists			
Pramipexole (Mirapex) (10,11)	0.125, 0.25, 0.5, 1.0, 1.5 mg tablets	7-week titration as needed to maximum dose of 4.5 mg/d to 0.125 tid; 0.25 tid; 0.5 tid; 0.75 tid; 1.0 tid; 1.25 tid; 1.5 tid	12% to 24%
Ropinirole (Requip) (12,13)	0.25, 0.5, 1.0, 2.0, 3.0, 4.0, 5.0 mg tablets	8-week titration: 0.25 tid; 0.5 tid; 0.75 tid; 1.0 tid; 1.5 tid; 2.0 tid; 2.5 tid; 3.0 tid; increase as needed to maximum dose of 24 mg/d	7% to 19%
Ropinirole XL (Requip XL)	2, 4, 8 mg tablets	Start with 2 mg daily for first 1 to 2 weeks; increase to 4 mg daily week 3; weekly titration up by 2 mg as necessary to a maximum dose of 24 mg daily	
Apomorphine (Apokyn) (16)	3 mL cartridges to extract dose for subcutaneous injection	Use as needed; start with 0.2 mL (2 mg) and titrate by 0.1 or 0.2 mL increases as necessary to a maximum dose of 0.6 mL (6 mg)	34% 2.0 h
COMT inhibitors			
Entacapone (Comtan) (8,17)	200 mg tablets	200 mg with each dose of levodopa up to 8 times per day, not to exceed 1600 mg/d of entacapone	12% to 22% 0.7 to 1.2 h
Carbidopa/ levodopa/ entacapone (Stalevo 50, 100, 150, 200)	12.5/50/200, 25/100/200, 37.5/150/200, 50/200/200 mg tablets	Replace each levodopa dose up to a maximum of 1600 mg/d entacapone or 1200 mg/d levodopa	See data for entacapone above
Tolcapone (Tasmar) (18,19)	100 mg, 200 mg tablets	Start with 100 mg tid and increase to 200 mg tid as necessary	12% to 28% 0.9 to 1.8 h

Table 7.3 *continued*

Amantadine			
Amantadine (Symmetrel) (20)	100 mg tablets	Start with 100 mg and increase to 100 bid or tid	Insufficient data
Deep brain stimulation			
Subthalamic nucleus (22)	Unilateral or bilateral	Data based on bilateral procedures	58% to 79%

[a] corrected for placebo effect and based on pivotal trials or highest class of evidence published; bid, twice daily; qd, once daily; tid, three times daily.

Table 7.4 Guidelines for the treatment of motor fluctuations in advanced Parkinson's disease

Treatment	AAN (2006)[4]	MDS (2005)[5]	EFNS (2006)[6]
MAO-B inhibitors			
Rasagiline (Azilect)	Effective	Insufficient data	Recommended
Orally disintegrating selegiline (Zelapar)	Possibly effective	Not discussed	Recommended
Selegiline (Eldepryl)	Possibly effective	Insufficient data	Inconsistent data
Dopamine agonists			
Pramipexole (Mirapex)	Probably effective	Effective; clinically useful	Recommended
Ropinirole (Requip)	Probably effective	Effective; clinically useful	Recommended
Rotigotine (Neupro)	Not discussed	Not discussed	Not discussed
Apomorphine (Apokyn)	Possibly effective	Effective; clinically useful	Recommended
COMT inhibitors			
Entacapone (Comtan)	Effective	Effective; clinically useful	Recommended
Tolcapone (Tasmar)	Probably effective	Effective; possibly useful	Recommended
Amantadine (dyskinesia; insufficient data for "off" time)			
Amantadine (Symmetrel)	Possibly effective	Effective; clinically useful	Recommended
Deep brain stimulation (motor fluctuations and dyskinesia)			
Thalamus	Insufficient data	Insufficient data	Not recommended
Globus pallidus	Insufficient data	Insufficient data	Not recommended
Subthalamic nucleus	Possibly effective	Insufficient data	Recommended

AAN, American Academy of Neurology; COMT, catechol-*O*-methyltransferase; EFNS, European Federation of Neurological Societies; MAO-B, monoamine oxidase type B; MDS, Movement Disorder Society.

can be increased to reduce off time at the risk of causing dyskinesia and, similarly, it can be decreased to reduce dyskinesia at the risk of increasing off time. Due to the difficulty in balancing motor fluctuations and dyskinesia with levodopa adjustments, the use of additional agents may be more beneficial in some patients.[1]

Immediate-release levodopa can be replaced with an extended-release formulation of levodopa to reduce off time.[1] The bioavailability of extended-release levodopa is less than that of the immediate-release formulation, so the dose may need to be increased by 20% to 30%. Alternatively, a treatment regimen utilizing both immediate- and extended-release preparations could be used depending upon the pattern of off time. However, several studies have compared immediate- and extended-release levodopa and have found no differences in off time, dyskinesia, or adverse events.[4]

MAO-B inhibitors

MAO-B inhibitors increase the amount of levodopa that reaches the brain by inhibiting the metabolism of dopamine by the MAO enzyme. MAO-B inhibitors currently available in the United States are rasagiline (Azilect), selegiline (Eldepryl), and orally disintegrating selegiline (Zelapar). These are all selective, irreversible inhibitors of MAO-B; however, at higher than recommended doses, these medications may also inhibit MAO-A. Several drugs are contraindicated with MAO-B inhibitors, including other MAO inhibitors; analgesics such as meperidine (Demerol), methadone (Dolophine, Methadose), and propoxyphene (Darvon); dextromethorphan; mirtazapine (Remeron); cyclobenzaprine (Flexeril); sympathomimetic amines including amphetamines and cold or weight-loss products containing vasoconstrictors; and St. John's wort.

Rasagiline

Rasagiline is a once-daily preparation approved as monotherapy and as an adjunct treatment to levodopa. It is rapidly absorbed and has a half-life of about 3 hours. In advanced disease, rasagiline is started at 0.5 mg once a day and is increased to 1.0 mg once a day if necessary. In a 26-week, double-blind, placebo-controlled study of PD subjects with motor fluctuations, rasagiline 0.5 mg/day decreased daily off time by 23% (1.4 hours), and rasagiline 1.0 mg/day decreased daily off time by 29% (1.9 hours), compared to a decrease of 15% (0.9 hours) with placebo.[7] In an 18-week study, rasagiline 1.0 mg/day reduced daily off time by 21% (1.2 hours), compared to a decrease of 7% (0.4 hours) with placebo.[8] This study also included an active comparator arm in which subjects received 200 mg of entacapone with each dose of levodopa. In this arm, there was also a 21% (1.2 hours) reduction in daily off time. The most common adverse events with rasagiline were dyskinesia, nausea, weight loss, constipation, postural hypotension, vomiting, dry mouth, rash, and somnolence.

Selegiline

Selegiline is approved as an adjunct treatment to levodopa. It is absorbed in the gastrointestinal tract and metabolized by the liver with a half-life of 2 hours. The recommended dose of selegiline is 5 mg at breakfast and lunch; doses after lunch are not recommended due to potential insomnia caused by its amphetamine metabolites. The AAN guidelines[4] recommend that selegiline may be considered to reduce off time; however, the MDS guidelines[5] concluded that there were insufficient data, and the EFNS guidelines[6] suggest that the current data are inconsistent. The most common adverse events with selegiline are nausea, dizziness, insomnia, confusion, hallucinations, constipation, orthostatic hypotension, dry mouth, and dyskinesia.

Orally disintegrating selegiline

Orally disintegrating selegiline is approved as an adjunct treatment to levodopa. This form of selegiline minimizes first-pass metabolism as it dissolves rapidly on the tongue and is absorbed through the buccal mucosa, which minimizes the amphetamine metabolites. It is initiated at 1.25 mg once a day and increased to 2.5 mg once a day after 6 weeks if necessary. In a 12-week, double-blind, placebo-controlled study of PD subjects with motor fluctuations, orally disintegrating selegiline decreased off time by 23% (2.2 hours per day), compared to 9% (0.6 hours per day) with placebo with a corresponding increase in on time without dyskinesia of 1.8 hours per day. The most common adverse events were dizziness, dyskinesia, hallucinations, headache, and dyspepsia.[9]

Dopamine agonists

Dopamine agonists do not require conversion to dopamine as they stimulate the postsynaptic dopamine receptors. Pergolide (Permax), an ergoline dopamine agonist, was removed from the U.S. market due to concerns of cardiac valvular fibrosis. Therefore, persons with past exposure to pergolide should receive echocardiogram screening. Due to concerns of ergoline-related adverse events, bromocriptine (Parlodel) is rarely used in clinical practice, and the AAN guidelines[4] concluded that it was not effective in reducing off time. Other dopamine agonists currently available in the United States are pramipexole (Mirapex), ropinirole (Requip), ropinirole XL (Requip XL), and apomorphine (Apokyn). Rotigotine (Neupro) was recently removed from the U.S. market due to manufacturing problems. Adverse events for these agonists include nausea, vomiting, dyskinesia, dizziness, somnolence, insomnia, pedal edema, orthostatic hypotension, hallucinations, confusion, mood changes, euphoria, vivid dreams, and sleep problems. There have also been reports of unexpected sleep episodes and impulsive behaviors such as gambling, shopping, sexual behaviors, and eating.

Pramipexole

Pramipexole is a nonergoline dopamine agonist approved as monotherapy and as an adjunct to levodopa. It acts primarily on the D2, D3, and D4 dopamine receptors and has a half-life of 8 to 12 hours. Pramipexole is initiated at 0.125 mg 3 times a day and increased slowly over 7 weeks to a maximum recommended dose of 1.5 mg 3 times a day (Table 7.3). A 32-week, double-blind, placebo-controlled study of PD subjects with motor fluctuations reported a 31% decrease in daily off time with pramipexole (up to

4.5 mg/day), compared to a 7% reduction with placebo.[10] In a similar study, pramipexole (mean 3.36 mg/day) was shown to reduce daily off time by 15% (2.5 hours), compared to 3% with placebo.[11]

Ropinirole

Ropinirole is a nonergoline dopamine agonist approved as monotherapy and as adjunctive therapy. It acts primarily on the D2 dopamine receptor family, with little action on D1 or D5 receptors, and has a half-life of about 6 hours. It is initiated at 0.25 mg 3 times a day and is slowly increased over 8 weeks to 3 mg 3 times a day, with further increases as needed to a maximum dose of 24 mg/day (Table 7.3). In a 24-week, double-blind, placebo-controlled study of PD subjects with motor fluctuations, ropinirole reduced daily off time by 11.7%, compared to 5.1% with placebo.[12] Similarly, in a 12-week, double-blind, placebo-controlled study of PD subjects with motor fluctuations, ropinirole (mean 6.6 mg/day) decreased daily off time by 23%, compared to 4% with placebo.[13]

Ropinirole XL (Requip XL) was recently approved for the treatment of PD. The effects of this 24-hour prolonged-release formulation of ropinirole on daily off time were examined in a 24-week, double-blind, placebo-controlled study of PD subjects with daily off time.[14] This once-daily formulation of ropinirole provides for faster titration compared to immediate-release ropinirole, with fewer adverse events. It was shown to reduce daily off time by 2.1 hours, compared to 0.3 hours with placebo, while significantly increasing on time without troublesome dyskinesia. Ropinirole XL is started at 2 mg once a day and increased by 2 mg every 1 to 2 weeks to a maximum dose of 24 mg per day.

Rotigotine

Rotigotine is a nonergoline dopamine agonist delivered through a transdermal system. The drug was recently removed from the U.S. market due to a manufacturing problem, but it is expected to be released again in the future. It acts primarily on the D3, D2, and D1 dopamine receptors and has some action on the D4 and D5 receptors. It is absorbed over 24 hours and has a half-life of 5 to 7 hours. The patch can be applied to various locations on the body and should be changed daily, avoiding application to the same site for at least 14 days to reduce skin irritation. Rotigotine is currently approved for the treatment of early PD at a maximum recommended dose of 6 mg every 24 hours and has also been shown to reduce motor complications in advanced PD.[15] In a 24-week, double-blind, placebo-controlled study of PD patients with daily off time, rotigotine 8 mg/24 hours reduced off time by 2.7 hours per day, and rotigotine 12 mg/24 hours by 2.1 hours per day, compared to a reduction of 0.9 hours per day with placebo. In addition, there was a significant increase in on time without troublesome dyskinesia with preparations of 8 mg and 12 mg/24 hours as compared to placebo. Adverse events were typical of other dopamine agonists except for skin reactions at the site of the patch, which occurred in 36% of the 8 mg/24hours group, 46% of the 12 mg/24 hours group and 13% of the placebo group. The majority of the skin reactions were mild, with only 3% reported to be severe.

Apomorphine

Apomorphine is injected subcutaneously and is a rescue therapy approved for advanced PD patients who experience off periods. It is a nonergoline, fast-acting dopamine agonist with affinity for all dopamine receptors. It is rapidly absorbed and takes effect in 10 to 60 minutes; it has a half-life of about 40 minutes and an action of up to 90 minutes. The initial dose is given under medical supervision, starting at 0.2 mL (2 mg) and titrated by 0.1 mL increments until an effective dose is obtained, not to exceed a single dose of 0.6 mL. It can be administered every 2 hours, but it is not recommended to exceed 5 daily doses. Apomorphine is an emetic and can cause severe nausea and vomiting; therefore, it is recommended that an antiemetic such as trimethobenzamide (Tigan) be used 3 days prior to and at least 6 weeks after initial administration. To avoid severe hypotension and potential loss of consciousness, apomorphine should not be used with 5HT3 antagonists such as ondansetron (Zofran). A double-blind, placebo-controlled study reported a decrease of 34% (2.0 hours per day) in off time with subcutaneous apomorphine, compared to no change with placebo.[16]

COMT inhibitors

Catechol-O-methyl transferase (COMT) inhibitors are used only in combination with levodopa, and they increase the amount of levodopa that reaches the brain by blocking the COMT enzyme, which breaks down levodopa. COMT inhibitors available in the United States are entacapone (Comtan), which is also available as a triple-combination formulation of carbidopa/levodopa/entacapone (Stalevo 50, 100, 150 and 200), and tolcapone (Tasmar). The most common adverse events are dyskinesia, nausea, vomiting, hallucinations, diarrhea, discoloration of urine, and dizziness.

Entacapone

Entacapone is approved for PD patients on levodopa with end-of-dose wearing-off. It has a half-life of about 30 minutes and increases the half-life of levodopa up to 2.4 hours. One 200 mg dose of entacapone is given with each dose of levodopa (up to 8 doses per day). An 18-week, double-blind, placebo-controlled study of PD patients with motor fluctuations reported a decrease in daily off time of 21% (1.2 hours) with entacapone, compared to 7% (0.4 hours) with placebo.[8] There was also a significant increase of 0.9 hours of daily on time without troublesome dyskinesia. In a similar, 24-week, double-blind, placebo-controlled study, entacapone decreased daily off time by 23.6% (1.3 hours), compared to 1.9% (0.1 hours) with placebo.[17]

Entacapone is also available in four strengths of a triple-combination with carbidopa and levodopa. The different strengths contain 200 mg of entacapone and 50, 100, 150, or 200 mg of levodopa, with a corresponding dose of carbidopa in a 1:4 ratio with levodopa (Table 7.3). The triple combination is approved as a substitute for carbidopa/levodopa and entacapone used separately, or in patients taking no more than 200 mg of levodopa in each single dose who are experiencing end-of-dose wearing-off. The total daily dose should not exceed 1600 mg of entacapone or 1200 mg of levodopa. Safety and efficacy are similar to carbidopa/levodopa and entacapone used separately.

Tolcapone

Tolcapone is approved as an adjunct to levodopa. It has a half-life of 2 to 3 hours and is initiated at 100 mg 3 times a day, with an increase to 200 mg 3 times a day if needed. In a 12-week, double-blind, placebo-controlled study of PD patients with wearing off, daily off time was reduced by tolcapone 100 mg 3 times a day by 32% (2.3 hours) and by tolcapone 200 mg 3 times a day by 48% (3.2 hours), compared to a reduction of 20% (1.4 hours) by placebo.[18] In a similar 12-week study, tolcapone 100 mg 3 times a day reduced off time by 31.5%, tolcapone 200 mg 3 times a day by 26.2%, and placebo by 11%.[19] Due to three cases of fatal liver damage with tolcapone, liver enzyme testing should be done every 2 to 4 weeks for the first 6 months and as clinically indicated thereafter.

Amantadine

Amantadine is an antiviral agent, and its exact mechanism of action in PD is unknown. It is quickly absorbed, reaches peak plasma levels in 2 to 4 hours, and should be used with caution in persons with renal disease. The most common dose is 200 to 300 mg/day in divided doses. A double-blind, placebo-controlled, crossover study of 24 PD subjects found a 24% reduction in dyskinesia with amantadine.[20] Another double-blind, placebo-controlled study found a decrease in dyskinesia of 45%; however, these effects were only maintained for approximately 8 months.[21] Adverse events with amantadine include dizziness, insomnia, anxiety, nausea, vomiting, pedal edema, and livedo reticularis.

Other therapies

Deep brain stimulation

When medications can no longer control motor complications, deep brain stimulation (DBS) may be an option. DBS is currently the most commonly used surgical treatment for PD and involves a DBS electrode placed in the brain and connected to an implantable pulse generator (IPG). The IPG is the power source or battery of the system and is generally placed in the chest.[22] In the treatment of PD, the stimulating electrode can be placed in the thalamus, globus pallidus (GPi), or subthalamic nucleus (STN). The latter is currently the most common surgical target for PD. DBS of the thalamus has not been shown to significantly affect motor complications, and, according to the AAN guidelines, there are currently insufficient data on the effects of GPi DBS on motor complications.[4] However, STN DBS has been shown to be successful in reducing both motor fluctuations and dyskinesia. A meta-analysis of the DBS literature indicated that STN DBS reduced off time by an average of 68.2% and reduced dyskinesia by an average of 69.1%, effects which have been shown to be maintained for at least 5 years.[22]

Candidates for STN DBS include idiopathic PD patients with a good response to levodopa who are experiencing motor complications without significant cognitive, behavioral, psychiatric, or other medical conditions. Serious adverse events related to the surgical procedure include hemorrhage, stroke, or seizures (which are uncommon, occurring in less than 1% to 2% of patients) and infection, which is reported in approximately 5% to 7% of patients. Adverse events related to the stimulation are generally mild and resolve with adjustments of stimulation parameters. Device-related adverse events include breakage or malfunction of the DBS components and occur in 10% to 25% of patients. The battery is replaced every 3 to 5 years as an outpatient procedure.[23]

Conclusion

The management of a PD patient with motor disability depends on whether motor complications are present. If the patient has motor fluctuations and is currently on levodopa alone, the options include increasing the dosage or frequency of levodopa; using adjunctive therapy with MAO-B inhibitors, dopamine agonists, or COMT inhibitors; or switching to extended-release levodopa preparations. The decision about which strategy to employ is based on the individual characteristics and symptoms of the patient. Eventually, a patient may receive combination therapy using several or all of the adjunctive therapies. If the patient's main problem is dyskinesia, the options include reducing levodopa or adjunctive therapies or adding amantadine. If motor complications cannot be managed with medications, deep brain stimulation may be an option. If the main problems include freezing of gait or postural instability, medications are usually not helpful and physical therapy should be tried. In some patients with freezing or postural instability who are at risk for frequent falls, a wheelchair or motorized scooter may be necessary.

References

1. Olanow CW, Watts RL, Koller WC. An algorithm (decision tree) for the management of Parkinson's disease (2001): treatment guidelines. *Neurology.* 2001;56(11 suppl 5):S1–S88.

2. Chapuis S, Ouchchane L, Metz O, Gerbaud L, Durif F. Impact of the motor complications of Parkinson's disease on the quality of life. *Mov Disord.* 2005;20(2):224–230.

3. Schrag A, Ben-Shlomo Y, Brown R, Marsden CD, Quinn N. Young-onset Parkinson's disease revisited—clinical features, natural history, and mortality. *Mov Disord.* 1998;13(6):885–894.

4. Pahwa R, Factor SA, Lyons KE, et al. Practice parameter: treatment of Parkinson disease with motor fluctuations and dyskinesia (an evidence-based review): report of the Quality Standards Subcommittee of the American Academy of Neurology. *Neurology.* 2006;66(7):983–995.

5. Goetz CG, Poewe W, Rascol O, Sampaio C. Evidence-based medical review update: pharmacological and surgical treatments of Parkinson's disease: 2001 to 2004. *Mov Disord.* 2005;20(5):523–539.

6. Horstink M, Tolosa E, Bonuccelli U, et al. Review of the therapeutic management of Parkinson's disease. Report of a joint task force of the European Federation of Neurological Societies (EFNS) and the Movement Disorder Society-European Section (MDS-ES). Part II: late (complicated) Parkinson's disease. *Eur J Neurol.* 2006;13(11):1186–1202.

7. Parkinson Study Group. A randomized placebo-controlled trial of rasagiline in levodopa-treated patients with Parkinson disease and motor fluctuations: the PRESTO study. *Arch Neurol.* 2005;62(2):241–248.

8. Rascol O, Brooks DJ, Melamed E, et al. Rasagiline as an adjunct to levodopa in patients with Parkinson's disease and motor fluctuations (LARGO, Lasting effect in Adjunct therapy with Rasagiline Given Once daily, study): a randomised, double-blind, parallel-group trial. *Lancet.* 2005;365(9463):947–954.

9. Waters CH, Sethi KD, Hauser RA, Molho E, Bertoni JM. Zydis selegiline reduces off time in Parkinson's disease patients with motor fluctuations: a 3-month, randomized, placebo-controlled study. *Mov Disord.* 2004;19(4):426–432.

10. Lieberman A, Ranhosky A, Korts D. Clinical evaluation of pramipexole in advanced Parkinson's disease: results of a double-blind, placebo-controlled, parallel-group study. *Neurology.* 1997;49(1):162–168.

11. Guttman M. Double-blind comparison of pramipexole and bromocriptine treatment with placebo in advanced Parkinson's disease. International Pramipexole-Bromocriptine Study Group. *Neurology.* 1997;49(4):1060–1065.

12. Lieberman A, Olanow CW, Sethi K, et al. A multicenter trial of ropinirole as adjunct treatment for Parkinson's disease. Ropinirole Study Group. *Neurology.* 1998;51(4):1057–1062.

13. Rascol O, Lees AJ, Senard JM, Pirtosek Z, Montastruc JL, Fuell D. Ropinirole in the treatment of levodopa-induced motor fluctuations in patients with Parkinson's disease. *Clin Neuropharmacol.* 1996;19(3):234–245.

14. Pahwa R, Stacy MA, Factor SA, et al. Ropinirole 24-hour prolonged release: randomized, controlled study in advanced Parkinson disease. *Neurology.* 2007;68(14):1108–1115.

15. LeWitt PA, Lyons KE, Pahwa R. Advanced Parkinson disease treated with rotigotine transdermal system: PREFER study. *Neurology.* 2007;68(16):1262–1267.

16. Dewey RB Jr., Hutton JT, LeWitt PA, Factor SA. A randomized, double-blind, placebo-controlled trial of subcutaneously injected apomorphine for parkinsonian off-state events. *Arch Neurol.* 2001;58(9):1385–1392.

17. Rinne UK, Larsen JP, Siden A, Worm-Petersen J. Entacapone enhances the response to levodopa in parkinsonian patients with motor fluctuations. Nomecomt Study Group. *Neurology.* 1998;51(5):1309–1314.

18. Rajput AH, Martin W, Saint-Hilaire MH, Dorflinger E, Pedder S. Tolcapone improves motor function in parkinsonian patients with the "wearing-off" phenomenon: a double-blind, placebo-controlled, multicenter trial. *Neurology.* 1997;49(4):1066–1071.

19. Baas H, Beiske AG, Ghika J, et al. Catechol-O-methyltransferase inhibition with tolcapone reduces the "wearing off" phenomenon and levodopa requirements in fluctuating parkinsonian patients. *J Neurol Neurosurg Psychiatry.* 1997;63(4):421–428.

20. Snow BJ, Macdonald L, McAuley D, Wallis W. The effect of amantadine on levodopa-induced dyskinesias in Parkinson's disease: a double-blind, placebo-controlled study. *Clin Neuropharmacol.* 2000;23(2):82–85.

21. Thomas A, Iacono D, Luciano AL, Armellino K, Di Iorio A, Onofrj M. Duration of amantadine benefit on dyskinesia of severe Parkinson's disease. *J Neurol Neurosurg Psychiatry.* 2004;75(1):141–143.

22. Kleiner-Fisman G, Herzog J, Fisman DN, et al. Subthalamic nucleus deep brain stimulation: summary and meta-analysis of outcomes. *Mov Disord.* 2006;21 (suppl 14):S290–S304.

23. Lyons KE, Pahwa R. Deep brain stimulation in Parkinson's disease. *Curr Neurol Neurosci Rep.* 2004;4(4):290–295.

Chapter 8

Management of nonmotor manifestations of Parkinson's disease

Benzi M. Kluger and Hubert H. Fernandez

Although Parkinson's disease (PD) is traditionally thought of as a disorder of motor function, nonmotor symptoms are increasingly recognized as a significant source of disability and suffering. Nonmotor symptoms can be classified as intrinsic or iatrogenic. The most common intrinsic nonmotor symptoms recognized in PD patients are depression, cognitive impairment, sleep disorders, and autonomic dysfunction. Frequent iatrogenic complications include psychosis, compulsions, and impulse control disorders. These symptoms often do not respond to standard dopaminergic PD therapies. In fact, dopaminergic medications frequently contribute to the onset and exacerbation of these symptoms. The spectrum of nonmotor manifestations of PD is reviewed in Chapter 1. This chapter highlights some of the unique challenges associated with their treatment.

Management of depression in PD

Although the prevalence of clinically significant depression in PD may be as high as 45%, it is often not recognized by clinicians.[1] In part, this may be because many of the cardinal symptoms of PD are similar to depressive symptoms, such as masked facies, disrupted sleep, weight loss, and psychomotor retardation. Additionally, PD patients with depression manifest fewer symptoms of sadness and guilt and more symptoms of decreased concentration and irritability compared to depressed patients without PD. Depression may start at any time during the progression of PD, and may even precede motor symptoms. It is not correlated to the degree of motor severity in PD. Depression is important to treat, as it is related to poor quality of life for both the patient and the caregiver.

As in other populations, it is important to rule out secondary causes of depression before proceeding to pharmacological treatments. This workup may include a complete blood count, liver function tests, serum testosterone levels, and thyroid function tests. It is important to review current medications, as many drugs can have depressive side effects. A unique point to pursue with the PD patient is whether the depressive symptoms relate to motor fluctuations or the timing of PD medications. Depressive symptoms may be a nonmotor manifestation of an "off" state in some patients and may be improved by smoothing out these fluctuations.

There is a paucity of data concerning the use of specific antidepressants in treating depression in PD. Recently published practice parameters on the management of depression in PD note that while a single class II study suggests that amitriptyline may be superior to selective serotonin reuptake inhibitors (SSRIs), there is currently insufficient evidence to evaluate the efficacy of other antidepressants, and so amitriptyline may not be the first choice for many patients. The side-effect profiles of these medications may guide in the selection of a particular treatment (Table 8.1). While SSRIs are generally better tolerated than tricyclic antidepressants (TCAs), there are certain situations in which TCAs may be preferred. Tertiary amine TCAs (amitriptyline, imipramine, and doxepin) may be beneficial in patients with insomnia, bladder hyperactivity, and drooling, because of their anticholinergic effects. In contrast, these anticholinergic properties may worsen cognitive impairment, hallucinations, hypotension, or excessive daytime somnolence. Depressed patients with comorbid anxiety may also respond better to SSRIs.

Other medications that have been found to be effective in the treatment of depression in PD include nefazodone, mirtazapine, and dopamine agonists (DAs). Both nefazodone and mirtazapine may be useful in patients with concomitant insomnia. The DA pramipexole has shown efficacy in treating depression in patients with and without PD. A recent randomized controlled trial (RCT) demonstrated that pramipexole had a significantly higher response rate than sertraline in treating depression in PD, though investigators used low-dose sertraline.[2] Studies have also found that ropinirole improves depression as a secondary outcome in PD. Finally, certain medications should be avoided in the patient with PD. Amoxapine and lithium both have the potential to cause or worsen parkinsonism, and nonselective monoamine oxidase inhibitors can lead to a hypertensive crisis in PD patients on levodopa.

Nonpharmacological treatments for depression in PD include cognitive-behavioral therapy (CBT) and electroconvulsive therapy (ECT). CBT has shown efficacy as an add-on or stand-alone treatment in major depression. A recent pilot study suggests that CBT may be effective in PD.[3] Although there have been no RCTs of ECT as a treatment for depression in PD, several large series have shown that it is efficacious in PD and may help motor symptoms.[4] ECT should be reserved for patients who are refractory to medical treatment.

Transcranial magnetic stimulation (TMS) is another emerging nonpharmacological treatment for depression. TMS devices have been approved for the treatment of depression in Israel and Canada, and the U.S. Food and Drug Administration is currently considering approval of a device in the United States. Studies suggest that depression in PD can be safely treated with TMS, although further trials are needed to determine the optimal candidates and treatment parameters.[5]

Table 8.1 Side effects of antidepressants used in PD

Drug	Dose (mg/day)	Sedation	Hypotension	Antimuscarinic effects	Sexual dysfunction	Weight gain
Fluoxetine	10 to 80	Negligible	Negligible	Negligible	Considerable	Mild
Fluvoxamine	50 to 300	Negligible	Negligible	Negligible	Moderate	Moderate
Paroxetine	20 to 50	Mild	Negligible	Mild	Severe	Moderate
Sertraline	25 to 100	Negligible	Negligible	Negligible	Moderate	Mild
Citalopram	10 to 60	Mild	Negligible	Mild	Moderate	Mild
Escitalopram	10 to 20	Mild	Negligible	Mild	Moderate	Mild
Amitriptyline	25 to 200	Considerable	Moderate	Considerable	Mild	Considerable
Doxepin	75 to 150	Moderate	Moderate	Considerable	Mild	Moderate
Imipramine	50 to 200	Moderate	Considerable	Moderate	Mild	Moderate
Desipramine	100 to 300	Mild	Mild	Mild	Negligible	Mild
Nortriptyline	50 to 150	Mild	Mild	Mild	Negligible	Mild
Bupropion	150 to 450	Negligible	Negligible	Mild	Negligible	Negligible
Mirtazapine	15 to 45	Moderate	Moderate	Mild	Moderate	Considerable
Nefazodone	300 to 600	Moderate	Moderate	Negligible	Mild	Negligible
Venlafaxine	75 to 375	Mild	Negligible	Mild	Considerable	Mild

Management of cognitive dysfunction

Cognitive dysfunction is common even in early PD and increases in prevalence with disease progression. The profile of cognitive dysfunction in PD differs from that in Alzheimer's disease (AD) and typically involves frontal-executive functions including motivation, complex decision making, verbal fluency, and mental flexibility. Frontal lobe functions are poorly assessed by the Mini Mental State Examination. Screening of PD patients for cognitive dysfunction should include measures of frontal lobe function.

Dementia is defined as cognitive dysfunction in more than one neuropsychological domain (e.g., memory, frontal-executive, visual-spatial, language) that is severe enough to impair the patient's ability to live independently. The incidence of PD dementia is 4% to 9% per year, and the prevalence ranges from 20% to 80%, depending on the sample population, the criteria used, and the length of follow-up.[6] Dementia in PD limits pharmacotherapy of cardinal PD symptoms by increasing the risk of dopamine-induced confusion, agitation, and hallucinations. Dementia also contributes to caregiver stress, poor quality of life, early nursing home placement, and mortality.

Significant cognitive difficulties, particularly early in the disease, may indicate a primary diagnosis other than PD such as diffuse Lewy body disease, corticobasal degeneration, progressive supranuclear palsy, vascular dementia, or fronto-temporal dementia with parkinsonism. A workup for treatable conditions should include a brain imaging study, a complete metabolic panel, thyroid studies, B_{12} level, and serological studies for syphilis and HIV. A careful review of the patient's medications, including nonprescription, is essential to exclude drug-induced causes of cognitive decline (especially involving anticholinergics and sedative agents). A precipitous decline in cognition may be an indicator of an acute insult such as infection (e.g., urinary tract infection or pneumonia) or even a social stressor, such as moving.

Cholinesterase inhibitors and memantine have been shown to slow the progression and improve the cognitive and behavioral profile in patients with AD and have been studied in PD. A large RCT of rivastigmine in PD dementia has demonstrated improvements in cognition, daily activities, and neuropsychiatric complications and was the basis for approval of the agent for treatment of PD-related dementia.[7] Smaller trials suggest that donepezil and galantamine may be effective in PD, but large studies of these agents are lacking. Tacrine is rarely used due to the risk of hepatotoxicity and frequent dosing. The most common side effects of all cholinesterase inhibitors are gastrointestinal (GI) distress (nausea, diarrhea, vomiting), fatigue, nightmares, insomnia, and muscle cramps. GI symptoms typically resolve with time and may be minimized by taking the medication with food. Increased tremor may also be seen but is typically mild and transient.

So far there have been no clinical trials of memantine in the treatment of dementia in PD. One small study has shown it to be safe in PD and suggests that it possibly improves parkinsonian symptoms.[8] Side effects of memantine include headache, constipation, and confusion.

Management of impulse control disorders and compulsive behaviors

Impulse control disorders (ICD) are a set of pathological behaviors characterized by a failure to resist an impulse to perform acts that may have significant personal, familial, or financial consequences. Examples of ICD seen in PD include pathological gambling, hypersexuality, compulsive shopping, excessive spending, and binge eating. Compulsive behaviors, on the other hand, are characterized by repetitive behaviors that are often time-consuming or disruptive to the patient's normal routine. Examples include compulsive use of dopaminergic medications and "punding," a stereotyped motor behavior in which there is an intense fascination with repetitive handling and examining of mechanical objects, such as taking apart and reassembling appliances or sorting objects, such as pebbles. While each of these behaviors may be rare, collectively they may affect up to 6% of all PD patients and 14% of those taking DAs.[9] ICD and compulsive behaviors can lead to serious health conditions (compulsive eating, hypersexuality), large financial losses (gambling, shopping), and isolation from family members (punding). The risk of ICDs is higher with the use of DAs compared to other PD medications.

Management of these behaviors typically includes decreasing or discontinuing DA therapy (for ICD), lowering the overall dosage of PD medications, or the addition of an atypical antipsychotic drug (for compulsive behavior). However, there have been a few reports of punding becoming worse with quetiapine use.[10] Occasionally, clomipramine and other SSRIs may alleviate punding. Referrals for specific treatments (e.g., gambling counseling) or the use of behavioral interventions may also be helpful.

Management of sleep dysfunction and excessive daytime sleepiness

Sleep disorders affect 60% to 98% of PD patients.[11] The etiology of sleep disturbances in PD is often multifactorial and may arise as a primary manifestation of PD or secondary to medications, motor disturbances, pain, nocturia, cognitive problems, hallucinations, depression, and anxiety. Patients with PD may also be at higher risk for other common causes of sleep disturbance including restless legs syndrome (RLS), central and obstructive sleep apnea, periodic leg movements of sleep (PLMS), and rapid eye movement behavior disorder (RBD).

Given the number of conditions that can interfere with sleep, it is essential to take a complete history. It is important to determine whether patients are having difficulty with sleep initiation or sleep maintenance, as each may have different causes. Other important points to address include changes of PD symptoms during sleeping and waking hours, history of cognitive problems (sundowning, nocturnal hallucinations), motor disturbances (nocturnal akinesia, dyskinesias, painful dystonias), abnormal behaviors (nocturnal vocalizations, nightmares, dream enactment, leg movements), and urinary problems (nocturia). The spouse or caregiver should be asked about the patient's sleep, particularly regarding snoring and movements during sleep. A sleep diary, reflecting the hours of sleep and timing of medication dosages, is often helpful. An overnight sleep study may be necessary in determining a diagnosis and directing treatment.

Appropriate dosages of dopaminergic medication at bedtime may help relieve nocturnal akinesia, rigidity, pain, early morning dystonia, and wearing-off symptoms that can result in improved sleep. Controlled-release preparations are superior to immediate-release levodopa for decreasing sleep disturbances.[12] However, excessive nocturnal dopaminergic medication can lead to nocturnal dyskinesia and confusion, which can also interfere with sleep. Similarly, adequate treatment of depression and anxiety may improve sleep.

RLS occurs in approximately 20% of the PD population.[13] Patients should be tested for iron deficiency before initiating any treatment, as symptoms may resolve with adequate iron supplementation. PLMS is a distinct diagnosis that occurs in up to one-third of PD patients and is characterized by rhythmic movements of the extremities, mainly during non-REM sleep. RLS and PLMS frequently occur simultaneously, and their treatment can be similar. DAs taken 30 to 60 minutes before bedtime are the treatment of choice for RLS. Alternative treatments include controlled-release levodopa, clonazepam, gabapentin, and opiates.

RBD is characterized by vigorous (and sometimes injurious) behavior in REM sleep that usually represents enactment of vivid, action-filled, and/or violent dreams. The usual loss of muscle tone that is associated with normal REM sleep does not occur in RBD. In many cases RBD precedes the parkinsonian diagnosis, and one-third to half of RBD patients will develop PD or other types of α-synucleinopathy. Low-dose clonazepam (starting with 0.5 to 1 mg at bedtime) is the most effective drug for the treatment of RBD. Melatonin has also been reported to be effective, and potentially better tolerated, but no RCTs are available for either agent.[14] If a secondary cause of sleep disturbance is not found, clinicians may consider pharmacological treatments. The use of hypnotics (including over-the-counter preparations) should be approached cautiously, as these formulations can cause nocturnal confusion and daytime cognitive dysfunction. Daily use of these medications may also disrupt sleep and lead to withdrawal symptoms or rebound insomnia.

Excessive daytime sleepiness (EDS) affects 15% to 50% of patients with PD[15] and does not always correlate with the degree of nocturnal sleep disturbances. Reasons for EDS in PD are multifactorial and include involvement of the reticular activating system in the PD neurodegenerative process, PD motor dysfunction, depression, and side effects of dopaminergic medications. Dopaminergic treatments at low dosages may be sedating and induce sleep, whereas high dosages may paradoxically prolong sleep latency and disrupt sleep. Practitioners should also be aware that dopaminergic therapy, specifically DAs, may be associated with sudden-onset sleep ("sleep attacks"), which may lead to motor vehicle accidents. Patients should be alerted to this risk when starting these medications. These symptoms resolve after the responsible DA is discontinued.

For patients with EDS who do not have treatable sleep pathology or other secondary causes, stimulant medications given early in the day may be helpful. Modafinil has been shown to be effective in PD-related EDS. Short naps (15 to 30 minutes) may also be helpful in patients with EDS but should not be taken too late in the day, as they may then interfere with nocturnal sleep. See Table 8.2 for a summary of sleep disorders and their treatment.

Table 8.2 **Management of sleep disturbances in PD**

Sleep disturbance	Nonpharmacological management	Pharmacological treatments
Nocturnal PD symptoms (dystonia, rigidity, etc.)	Reduce nightly dose of dopaminergic medications (for nocturnal dyskinesia)	Nocturnal dose of continuous-release carbidopa/levodopa (for all other symptoms)
Restless legs syndrome Periodic leg movements during sleep	Iron supplementation Folate	Dopamine agonist qhs
		May also consider carbidopa/levodopa qhs, opiates, gabapentin, clonazepam
REM sleep behavior disorder	Ensure safety of sleep environment for patient and spouse	Clonazepam: start 0.5 mg qhs, may increase to 1 to 2 mg
		May also consider other benzodiazepines, melatonin
Excessive daytime sleepiness	Scheduled naps, exercise	Methylphenidate: start 5 mg daily
		Amantadine, 100 mg bid
		Modafinil, 50 to 100 mg qd
		Note: Do NOT take these medications after dinner
Obstructive sleep apnea	Weight loss	Positive pressure airway ventilation (CPAP/BiPAP)
Depression	Cognitive-behavioral therapy	Antidepressants, particularly mirtazapine, nefazodone, and TCAs
Nocturia	Restrict fluids before bedtime, bedside commode	Medications for the control of neurogenic bladder TCAs[a]
Hallucinations	Decrease dopaminergic medications	Quetiapine 12.5 to 50 mg qhs
Primary insomnia	Review good sleep hygiene	Cautious use of hypnotics

[a] See Table 8.3. bid, twice a day; BiPAP, bilevel positive airways pressure; CPAP, continuous positive airway pressure; qd, every day; qhs, at bedtime; qid, 4 times a day; TCA, tricyclic antidepressant.

Management of autonomic dysfunction

The autonomic nervous system is intrinsically involved in the neuropathology of PD. Over the course of PD, more than 90% of patients experience symptoms of autonomic dysfunction, which often results in a negative impact on quality of life. Autonomic symptoms seen in PD patients include orthostatic hypotension, dysfunctional bladder control, erectile dysfunction, diaphoresis, and GI symptoms.

Orthostatic hypotension is quite common in PD, affecting 20% to 50% of patients.[16] It is defined as a drop in systolic blood pressure of >20 mmHg or a decrease in diastolic pressure of >10 mmHg within 3 minutes of standing or head-up tilt. When orthostatic hypotension is diagnosed, medications that lower blood pressure must first be reduced or eliminated. It is not uncommon for patients with a history of hypertension to develop low blood pressure after being diagnosed with PD, thus requiring reduction of antihypertension medications. Dopaminergic medications (particularly DAs) may also aggravate orthostatic hypotension. Nonpharmacological strategies that may improve orthostatic symptoms include increasing fluid intake, increasing dietary salt, caffeine, and thigh-high support stockings. Raising the head of a bed 10 to 30 degrees may improve standing blood pressure and reduce risk of supine hypertension. If needed, pharmacological agents to raise blood pressure may be used. Midodrine is an α-1 agonist that should not be given later than 6:00 p.m. to avoid nocturnal hypertension. Fludrocortisone is a mineralocorticoid that works by volume expansion but which may lead to pedal or even pulmonary edema. Physostigmine, erythropoetin, and octreotide have also been reported to be useful.

Urinary symptoms associated with PD include nocturia, daytime polyuria, urinary urgency, and urge incontinence. It is important to recognize that other factors can contribute to urinary disturbances in the elderly, such as benign prostatic hypertrophy (BPH) in men and pelvic floor weakness in women. A complete urological evaluation is essential to select the correct diagnosis and treatment. Fluid intake should be reduced at night. Medications often used to treat urinary frequency, urgency, and stress incontinence are shown in Table 8.3. Most of these drugs should be used cautiously in men with BPH because of the possibility of bladder outlet obstruction. These medications also can exacerbate cognitive impairment, although trospium chloride may have fewer CNS effects. A bedside commode may be necessary if nocturia persists, particularly in patients at risk for falls.

Problems related to the GI system include sialorrhea, dysphagia, poor gastric motility, changes in appetite, constipation, and weight loss. Sialorrhea is more likely the result of decreased swallowing than of salivary overproduction. Unfortunately, anticholinergic drugs that are often used to relieve excessive drooling can easily cause confusion and worsen cognitive impairment. Botulinum toxin has been reported to alleviate sialorrhea in PD.[17] Nonpharmacological strategies include sucking sugar-free candies or chewing sugarless gum. Factors contributing to constipation include decreased

Table 8.3 Treatment of autonomic dysfunction in PD

Symptom	Nonpharmacological management	Pharmacological treatments
Orthostatic hypotension	Taper or discontinue unnecessary hypotensive drugs	Fludrocortisone, 0.1 mg qd
	Elevate head of bed 10 to 30 degrees	Midodrine, 5 to 10 mg tid; last dose before 6:00 pm to avoid supine hypertension
	Increase dietary salt (add salt tablets) and fluid intake	Ephedrine, 25 to 50 mg q 4 to 6 hours
	Thigh-high, fitted compression stockings	Phenylpropanolamine, start 25 mg bid *or* ergotamine/caffeine tablets *Note:* Should not be taken after dinner to avoid insomnia and supine hypertension
	Education: avoid standing quickly, hot environments, straining-type exercises, etc.	Consider physostigmine, erythropoietin, or octreotide
Constipation	Add dietary bulk	Stool softeners (e.g., docusate sodium 50 to 200 mg po qd)
	Increase fluid intake	Osmotic laxatives (lactulose, milk of magnesia)
	Regular exercise, mineral/tap water enemas	Stimulant laxative (bisacodyl) 10 to 15 mg po qd; 10 mg per rectum qd; *or* 30 mL Fleet enema
Excessive drooling	Encourage voluntary swallowing of saliva	Trihexyphenidyl 2 to 5 mg tid
	Sugar-free gum/hard candy	Benztropine 0.5 to 1.0 mg tid
		Glycopyrrolate 1 to 2 mg tid/qid
		Botulinum toxin type A or B, injection into parotid and submandibular salivary glands
Erectile dysfunction		Sildenafil 50 to 100 mg, Vardenafil 5 to 20 mg, or Tadalafil 5 to 20 mg 1 hour prior to intercourse; watch for orthostatic hypotension
		Yohimbine 5 to 10 mg tid
		Papaverine 1 to 4 mL of 30 mg/mL solution intracavernous injection
Urinary frequency (hyperactive bladder)		Tolterodine, 2 mg bid
		Oxybutynin, 5 mg tid/qid; patch q 3 days
		Propantheline, 15 to 30 mg qid

Table 8.3 *continued*

		Hyoscyamine, 0.15 to 0.3 mg qhs to qid
		Imipramine, 10 to 25 mg qhs
		Trospium chloride, 20 mg qhs
Urinary retention (hypoactive bladder)		Terazosin, start 1 mg qhs
		Doxazosin, 1 to 4 mg qd
		Prazosin, 1 mg bid to tid; may increase slowly up to 20 mg/day
		Tamsulosin, 0.4 to 0.8 mg qd
		Bethanechol chloride,
		10 to 50 mg po tid to qid;
		2.5 to 5 mg subcutaneously tid to qid
Drenching sweats/ diaphoresis	Prevent wearing-off symptoms at night	Carbidopa/levodopa CR qhs or addition of COMT inhibitor
		Propranolol, start 40 mg bid or 80 mg qd long-acting
		Clonidine, start with 0.1 mg/day

bid, twice a day; COMT, catechol-*O*-methyltransferase; CR, controlled release; po, orally; qd, every day; qhs, at bedtime; qid, 4 times a day; tid, 3 times a day.

physical activity, diminished intake of food and liquid, reduced force of abdominal muscle contractions, dysfunction of sphincters, and antiparkinsonian medications. Exercise, muscle conditioning, fiber, and medication use all play a role in combating constipation. Psyllium and stool softeners should be tried first to regulate bowel movement. If unsuccessful, lactulose can be added. Enemas, laxatives, or disimpaction may occasionally be needed to produce bowel movements.

Impotence and other forms of sexual dysfunction are probably underreported in PD. A thorough physical examination and urological assessment should be undertaken before treatment is initiated, as several potential causes of sexual dysfunction may be present, including depression, poor motor control, vascular disease, BPH, metabolic conditions, medications, and alcohol use. Occasionally, psychotherapy or the addition of levodopa at bedtime may improve symptoms. If not, urological consultation and the use of pharmacological agents may be considered.

If drenching sweats, especially at night, are part of an "off" phenomenon due to the long gap between the last dopaminergic dose at night and the first dose the next morning, adding sustained-release levodopa at bedtime may be considered. Propranolol or clonidine may be also used if PD medication adjustments do not relieve hyperhidrosis. See Table 8.3 for a summary of autonomic symptoms in PD and their treatment.

References

1. Shulman LM, Taback RL, Rabinstein AA, et al. Non-recognition of depression and other non-motor symptoms in Parkinson's disease. *Parkinsonism Relat Disord*. 2002;8(3):193–197.

2. Barone P, Scarzella L, Marconi R, et al. Pramipexole versus sertraline in the treatment of depression in Parkinson's disease: a national multicenter parallel-group randomized study. *J Neurol*. 253(5):601–607.

3. Dobkin RD, Allen LA, Menza M. Cognitive-behavioral therapy for depression in Parkinson's disease: a pilot study. *Mov Disord*. 2007;22(7):946–952.

4. Kennedy R, Mittal D, O'Jile J. Electroconvulsive therapy in movement disorders: an update. *J Neuropsychiatry Clin Neurosci*. 2003;15(4):407–421.

5. Fregni F, Pascual-Leone A. Transcranial magnetic stimulation for the treatment of depression in neurologic disorders. *Curr Psychiatry Rep*. 2005;7(5):381–390.

6. Breitner JC. Dementia—epidemiological considerations, nomenclature, and a tacit consensus definition. *J Geriatr Psychiatry Neurol*. 2006;19(3):129–136.

7. Aarsland D, Zaccai J, Brayne C. A systematic review of prevalence studies of dementia in Parkinson's disease. *Mov Disord*. 2005;20(10):1255–1263.

8. Merello M, Nouzeilles MI, Cammarota A, et al. Effect of memantine (NMDA antagonist) on Parkinson's disease: a double-blind crossover randomized study. *Clin Neuropharmacol*. 1999;22(5):273–276.

9. Fénelon G, Mahieux F, Huon R, et al. Hallucinations in Parkinson's disease: prevalence, phenomenology and risk factors. *Brain*. 2000;123(Pt 4):733–745.

10. Miwa H, Morita S, Nakanshi I, et al. Stereotyped behaviors or punding after quetiapine administration in Parkinson's disease. *Parkinsonism Relat Disord*. 2004; 10(3):177–180.

11. Thorpy MJ, Adler CH. Parkinson's disease and sleep. *Neurol Clin*. 2005;23(4): 1187–1208.

12. Pahwa R, Busenbark, Huber SJ, et al. Clinical experience with controlled-release carbidopa/levodopa in Parkinson's disease. *Neurology*. 1993;43(4):677–681.

13. Garcia-Borreguero D, Odin P, Serrano C. Restless legs syndrome and PD: a review of the evidence for a possible association. *Neurology*. 2003;61(6 suppl): 49–S55.

14. Boeve BF, Silber MH, Ferman TJ. Melatonin for treatment of REM behaviour disorders: results in 14 patients. *Sleep Med*. 2003;4(4):281–284.

15. Paus S, Brecht HM, Koster J, et al. Sleep attacks, daytime sleepiness, and dopamine agonists in Parkinson's disease. *Mov Disord*. 2003;18(6):659–667.

16. Pathak A, Senard JM. Blood pressure disorders during Parkinson's disease: epidemiology, pathophysiology and management. *Expert Rev Neurother*. 2006;6(8):173–1180.

17. Ondo WG, Hunter C, Moore W. A double-blind placebo-controlled trial of botulinum toxin B for sialorrhea in Parkinson's disease. *Neurology*. 2004; 62(1):7–40.

Chapter 9

Surgical management of Parkinson's disease

Ioannis U. Isaias and Michele Tagliati

Increasing interest in functional neurosurgery for Parkinson's disease (PD) has been fostered over the past decade by the limitations of levodopa therapy, our improved understanding of basal ganglia pathophysiology, and technological advances, most importantly the development of deep brain stimulation (DBS). When used for the treatment of movement disorders, DBS typically targets three areas of the brain: the ventral intermediate nucleus of the thalamus (Vim), the globus pallidus pars interna (GPi), and the subthalamic nucleus (STN). As Vim DBS almost exclusively improves contralateral tremor, it has been progressively replaced by DBS at the two other targets for PD treatment, even when tremor predominates.

Successful DBS therapy depends on the proper execution of several key steps, including accurate candidate selection, proper lead implant, competent programming, expert medication adjustments, and management of side effects. Postoperative management necessitates detailed knowledge of the anatomy and physiology of the target area, familiarity with programming protocols, and expertise in the pharmacological treatment of PD.

Selection criteria

The first and fundamental step of successful DBS therapy is proper patient selection. A retrospective analysis revealed that over 30% of patients labeled as "DBS failures" were simply not good candidates.[1] A diagnosis of idiopathic PD should be confirmed first, as DBS results in atypical parkinsonism have been disappointing. Patients with advanced PD complicated by motor fluctuations and dyskinesia despite best medication management should be considered for surgery, although there is no consensus on the specific degree of severity or Unified Parkinson Disease Rating Scale (UPDRS) score thresholds. The degree of preoperative change in UPDRS from medications off to medications on with levodopa challenge is considered the best predictor of outcome after DBS.[2]

Normal cognitive status should be established by proper neuropsychological testing,[3] as preoperative dementia is a risk factor for permanent cognitive decline after DBS. In addition, a psychiatric evaluation should assess the presence of untreated depression, anxiety, apathy, dopaminergic dysregulation syndrome, medication-induced hypomania/mania, psychotic symptoms, and suicide risk.[2] The role of age as outcome predictor for DBS is controversial. Advanced age has been correlated with negative outcomes such as cognitive decline and gait instability. Therefore, DBS candidates older than 70 years should be evaluated with particular care.

Finally, it is important for DBS candidates to have an educated, realistic view of what can be expected from the procedure. DBS is not a cure for PD and likely does not halt the progression of the disease. Optimal results may take months to achieve and may be different for each patient. An overview of selection criteria for DBS is summarized in Table 9.1.

Table 9.1 Selection criteria for deep brain stimulation (DBS) in patients with advanced Parkinson's disease (PD)

Selection criteria	Comment
Diagnosis of idiopathic PD	Atypical parkinsonism is generally unresponsive to DBS
Disease duration of 5 years or more	Atypical parkinsonism may initially manifest as PD, but will show atypical features within 3 to 5 years from onset
Good response to levodopa	Assessed either historically or with a levodopa challenge test (30% improvement or better)
Marked motor complications on dopaminergic therapy (e.g., severe dyskinesia, minimal "on" time without dyskinesia)	Level of disability may be interpreted differently by patient and physician; frequent drug administration cycles (q3h or less), severe dyskinesia, or prominent freezing responsive to levodopa should make DBS a consideration
Prominent refractory tremor	Disabling tremor unresponsive to levodopa may warrant DBS therapy even in the absence of severe motor fluctuations
Age range: 40 to 75 years	Older age is not a specific exclusion criteria; however, cognitive and general health status should be carefully evaluated in patients older than 70
Intact cognition	Cognitive impairment should be systematically ruled out, as worsening of cognitive status has been reported after DBS in patients with preexisting dementia
Absence of active psychiatric disease	Untreated psychiatric disease should be carefully addressed before considering DBS. Properly treated depression is not a contraindication but warrants careful post-surgical monitoring
Realistic expectations	DBS does not cure PD. Proper patient education is essential to ensure adequate expectations
Adequate social support	Patients with strong family or social support are better able to follow presurgical/surgical/post-surgical demands and show overall better outcomes

Surgical technique

Anatomic targeting: Neuroimaging techniques

Ventriculography is still utilized in several centers to locate the foramen of Monro and the anterior and posterior commissures. However, its importance is diminishing. Magnetic resonance imaging (MRI) is now widely used for targeting, due to its greater tissue resolution, no exposure to ionizing radiation, multiplanar imaging, and no visible artifact from compatible frames. The main disadvantage of MRI is the potential geometrical distortion introduced by nonlinearity of the magnetic field. The magnitude of distortion error in MRI appears to be sequence related. Fast spin-echo inversion-recovery imaging may be less susceptible to these magnetic distortions.

Physiological targeting: Recording techniques

Microelectrode recordings (MER) can accurately localize deep brain structures by recording individual neuronal activity. MER allows precise mapping of the target areas involved in movement and sensation. A potential disadvantage of microelectrode recordings is prolonged surgical time. However, target refinement with MER reduces the need to revise lead position due to incorrect anatomic targeting, which can occur in as many as 12% of cases.[1]

Implanting procedures

DBS implantation is usually performed in two stages. During the first stage, DBS leads are stereotactically implanted into the functional target. The decision of implanting staged unilateral or simultaneous bilateral leads is typically discussed on a case-by-case basis. In the author's experience, a staged implant may be particularly beneficial for older individuals (i.e., age >70 years), as it reduces the risk of postoperative confusion. The patient is awake in order to monitor neurological status and to facilitate physiological localization. The DBS lead is ≈1.3 mm in diameter and flexible, so that it moves with the brain and does not damage it. It is implanted and anchored to the skull with a burr hole "cap." A brain MRI is obtained immediately after surgery to confirm proper electrode placement and exclude hemorrhage. (A detailed description of this technique can be found in Ref. 4.)

During the second stage, which is performed under general anesthesia, the lead is connected subcutaneously to an implantable pulse generator (IPG), which is inserted beneath the skin of the chest wall. IPG implant is preferably performed 1 to 2 weeks after lead implant, allowing the brain to recover from bilateral frontal lobe penetrations before being subjected to a general anesthetic.

While frame-based targeting remains the gold standard for DBS lead placement, "frameless" techniques are gaining popularity.[5] The main advantage of these techniques is the enhancement of patient comfort through the elimination of the stereotactic frame. However, the accuracy of this technique remains unproven.

Postoperative management

A perfectly implanted lead in a well-selected patient is useless without the proper stimulation settings. Over one-third of patients referred to a specialized movement disorder center for "DBS failures" had not been properly programmed.[1] Primary goals of DBS programming are to maximize symptom suppression and minimize adverse effects. Minimizing battery drain and optimizing medication regimens are significant secondary goals.

The DBS device (Fig. 9.1) can be programmed to deliver stimulation in monopolar or bipolar configuration, employing any of the four contacts of a quadripolar lead, alone or in combination. Thus, a great deal of therapeutic flexibility is provided, permitting customized stimulation for each patient. Stimulation parameters can be adjusted at any time using a transcutaneous programmer.

In order to achieve these goals, one must take a systematic, multistep approach to DBS programming. Initial programming is usually postponed for about 2 to 4 weeks after surgery to allow for tissue healing and to prevent the microlesioning effect, which is the transient improvement of parkinsonian symptoms often observed after electrode implantation. The patient should be scheduled for a morning visit with medication withheld overnight or longer (practical off-drug condition). After recording impedance and current drain for each contact to assess device function, the therapeutic window of each contact is determined. This is the voltage range between the initial observation of reliable antiparkinsonian effects and the threshold for adverse events. The contact that yields the greatest antiparkinsonian effects or exhibits the greatest therapeutic window should be selected for chronic stimulation. Amplitudes between 2.5 and 3.5 V provide the best results in the majority of cases, in association with pulse widths in the 60 to 90 μs range and frequencies between 130 and 185 Hz.[6] If a single contact

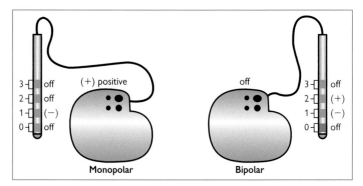

Figure 9.1 Deep brain stimulation device and most common programming configurations.

fails to provide satisfactory results, it may be useful to add another contact in order to broaden the effective field of stimulation. In certain situations, a bipolar setting can be used in order to achieve a more focused field of stimulation ("field shaping"). If no significant improvement is observed or stimulation-induced adverse events overwhelm clinical benefits, electrode position should be verified and technical troubleshooting begun.

The following key concepts should guide the assessment of stimulation clinical effects:

1. Rigidity is considered the most reliable symptom to evaluate, because it has a short latency to response time and is relatively stable as compared to tremor and bradykinesia.
2. Tremor is also a good target symptom, when it is present with an extremely short latency of response (usually a few seconds). However, tremor can be variable and influenced by the emotional state of the patient.
3. Bradykinesia has the longest latency of improvement, which may occur after several hours or even days.
4. Levodopa-induced dyskinesias can also be tremendously improved both by subthalamic and pallidal stimulation.[7] The effect of subthalamic DBS on dyskinesias is usually believed to be a byproduct of reduced levodopa requirements, but it has also been observed as a direct effect of stimulation, usually when the two most dorsal electrodes are activated.[8]

Before completing the first programming session, the patient should be observed after taking at least one standard dose of levodopa in order to address potential additive effects of medication and stimulation, including the onset of dyskinesias.

In general, the patient is sent home with the initial settings in monopolar configuration, using the contact with the best therapeutic window at the lowest effective voltage or slightly above. Over the next few weeks, however, a recurrence of parkinsonism is not uncommon, due either to further healing of the brain (with increased resistance to stimulation spread) or to the loss of the levodopa long-duration response secondary to medication reduction. Therefore, very cautious reduction or even no change of antiparkinsonian medications is advisable after initial programming. If parkinsonian symptoms reappear, adjustments of the initial parameters of stimulation are needed. The initial approach in adjusting DBS settings is to increase the amplitude of stimulation until an improvement comparable to the "on" levodopa state is observed.

The antiparkinsonian effect of STN DBS should, over time, approximate the benefits of levodopa therapy while eliminating or greatly reducing the associated motor fluctuations. As a consequence, dopaminergic medication can usually be reduced after STN DBS by 40% to 50%.[7,9] On rare occasions, some patients can even discontinue their pharmacological therapy. Pallidal and thalamic stimulation usually do not allow dramatic medication changes.

Results

The published experience with DBS for PD spans a period of almost 20 years. Positive results have been reported using all three main surgical targets for DBS implants.

Thalamus

High-frequency thalamic stimulation can efficiently suppress severe tremor in PD for several years after electrode implant. A large European study showed a significant reduction in contralateral upper and lower limb tremor in 85% of the patients. Akinesia and rigidity scores were moderately but significantly reduced, while axial scores were unchanged.[10] In a 5-year follow-up study of 19 PD patients, unilateral Vim implants yielded 85% improvement in targeted hand tremor while bilateral implants provided a virtual resolution of hand tremor.[11] However, Vim target is of limited use in PD due to lack of effect on the other PD symptoms.

Subthalamic nucleus

A large prospective, multicenter, double-blind, crossover study of STN DBS in 96 patients with advanced PD reported a mean improvement of 44% in UPDRS activities of daily living (ADL) scores and 51% in UPDRS motor scores.[9] Tremor improved dramatically (79%), but significant improvement in rigidity (58%), bradykinesia (42%), gait (56%), and postural instability (50%) were also observed. Most importantly, daily motor fluctuations were considerably reduced, with daily "off" time decreasing by 61%, "on" time increasing by 64%, and dyskinesias decreasing by 70%. A direct randomized comparison of STN DBS with best medical treatment in 156 patients with advanced PD resulted in a significant improvement in quality of life and motor function, with fewer dyskinesias compared to medications alone. Interestingly, the overall incidence of adverse events was higher in the medication arm.[12] A comprehensive meta-analysis of published STN DBS studies confirmed on a larger scale the postoperative symptomatic improvements and medication reductions previously described. According to this analysis, improvement after STN DBS was predicted by worse baseline severity, longer disease duration, and levodopa responsiveness.[13] Data on long-term outcomes of bilateral STN DBS in patients with advanced PD provide reassuring evidence for the stability of the results up to 5 years. However, STN DBS benefits seem to decline over time for axial signs (including gait, postural stability, and speech), as compared to a sustained improvement for tremor, bradykinesia, and rigidity. Finally, there is no evidence suggesting that STN DBS may affect the rate of progression of PD, although this topic is the object of current research.

Globus pallidum pars interna

Shortly after the initial experience with STN, satisfactory results for severe PD symptoms, motor fluctuations, and dyskinesias were reported using GPi DBS. The consistent effect of pallidal stimulation is a marked reduction of contralateral levodopa-induced dyskinesias. Improvement of "off-period" symptoms is also significant in most studies, in the range of 30% to 50%. A prospective, multicenter, double-blind, crossover study in 41 patients reported significant improvement of tremor, rigidity, bradykinesia, gait, and postural stability at 6 months.[9] Furthermore, dyskinesia-free "on" time was increased by about 35%, and "off" time was decreased by 13%.

Long-term studies with GPi stimulation have provided less consistent results. Return of dyskinesias and increased need of medication was reported in one study after 12 months, despite a residual 32% improvement in off-medication motor scores at 24 months.[14] In another series of PD patients followed for 5 years, the initial improvement of motor symptoms and fluctuations gradually declined after the first year of stimulation, while dyskinesia remained significantly reduced until the last assessment.[15] A third long-term follow-up study reported sustained improvements in UPDRS, motor, and ADL scores and dyskinesia, as well as on and off time after 4 years of pallidal DBS.[16] A large randomized study of GPi versus STN stimulation is ongoing.

Adverse events

Clinical adverse events observed in patients undergoing DBS are usually related to the surgical procedure, the implanted hardware, or the stimulation itself.

Procedure-related adverse events

The most important surgical complication of DBS surgery is an intra-parenchymal hemorrhage, with a risk reported in 1% to 5% of cases.[17] The incidence and most frequent location of misplaced leads, which may be implanted outside the target nucleus and even in the cerebral ventricles, is unknown. In a series of 41 patients referred for "DBS failures," the authors found that 19 (46%) had suboptimally placed electrodes.[1] Electrode misplacement can be diagnosed radiographically and should be revised as soon as possible in order to minimize patient discomfort.

Hardware-related adverse events

More common are the risks related to the implanted hardware, which have been reported with frequencies varying from 2.7% to 50% of patients. Infections after DBS implants have been reported with rates varying from 1% to 15%. In cases of active infection, hardware removal is strongly suggested, since attempts at providing antibiotic therapy without removal have a high rate of failure. A new IPG and extension cable can be replaced after 6 to 8 weeks of antibiotic therapy. Other hardware-related complications include electrode fracture, extension wire failure, lead migration, skin erosion, foreign body reaction, granuloma, seroma, IPG malfunction, and pain over the pulse generator.[17]

Stimulation-related adverse events

Thalamus

Adverse events in patients receiving unilateral thalamic implants include paresthesia and pain, while patients receiving bilateral implants complain mostly of dysarthria and balance difficulties. Other side effects include dysphagia, increased salivation, cognitive difficulties, and abnormal gait.[10] PD patients seem to experience tolerance (the reemergence of tremor after several months of effective stimulation) less frequently than patients with essential tremor.[18]

Subthalamic nucleus

Similar to thalamic DBS, dysarthria is probably the single most frequent adverse event interfering with successful subthalamic DBS in PD. It may be difficult to differentiate what is an adverse event related to stimulation and what is simply an unresolved or progressive symptom of the disease. Speech abnormalities are often unaffected by subthalamic DBS, yet specific speech difficulties that are temporally related to subthalamic stimulation are frequently encountered and are likely related to unwanted stimulation of corticobulbar fibers. Speech impairment secondary to stimulation is characterized subjectively by an increased effort to speak and objectively by hypophonia, hesitation, slurring of words, and rapid fatigue.[7] Careful adjustments of stimulation settings can prevent severe speech impairment in the vast majority of cases.

Occasionally, dysphagia is reported after successful STN programming. Similar to speech abnormalities, dysphagia can be a symptom of untreated PD, and only the temporal association with DBS suggests an etiologic correlation. Swallowing abnormalities may result from unwanted interference with signals carried to the swallowing muscles by corticobulbar fibers.

Another typical STN target-related adverse event is the development of dyskinesias, which are clinically similar to levodopa-induced dyskinesia and may, in fact, be worsened by levodopa therapy. Stimulation-induced dyskinesia can develop slowly over a period of minutes to hours[13] and can be managed with decreases in stimulation voltage and levodopa dose.

Postural instability is another symptom frequently encountered in patients with PD that can occasionally worsen or present de novo after subthalamic DBS. Preexisting postural instability that had previously responded to levodopa therapy is generally improved by subthalamic DBS.[19] Patients may complain of sensations of retropulsion and falls that were never experienced prior to DBS. In these instances, involvement of the cerebello-rubro-thalamic fibers medial to the STN or the red nucleus is postulated.[7] Decreasing stimulation energy and moving to more dorsal contacts or to bipolar configuration can improve balance.

Transient contralateral tingling sensations are usually predictive of good lead location and positive stimulation outcome. However, persistent paresthesias indicate current spread to the medial lemniscus or sensory thalamus. Decreasing stimulation amplitude and focusing the field with bipolar stimulation may relieve sensory symptoms. However, the presence of persistent dysesthesias at unusually low voltages should prompt consideration of lead revision.

A wide range of neuropsychiatric and cognitive complications of STN DBS surgery have been reported.[2,20] A large meta-analysis found cognitive problems in 41%, depression in 8%, and hypomania in 4% of the patients.

Anxiety disorders were observed in less than 2%, and personality changes, hypersexuality, apathy, anxiety, and aggressiveness were observed in less than 0.5% of the reported cases. About half of the patients did not experience behavioral changes.[21] Transient acute depression has been reported during STN DBS and may be related to stimulation of the substantia nigra.[22] In these cases, using more dorsal contacts will avoid this dramatic adverse event.

Diplopia, blurred vision, and abnormal eye movements are occasionally observed. These are not symptoms normally seen in PD and clearly suggest current diffusion toward the fibers of the oculomotor nerve, which sweep medially, ventrally, and posteriorly to the STN. In these cases, it is imperative to switch to a more dorsal contact and eventually lower the amplitude or change the configuration to bipolar (field shaping). If abnormal eye movements are observed at unusually low voltages, lead revision should be considered.

Globus pallidum pars interna

Complications of pallidal stimulation are less common.[14–16] Based on the anatomic proximity with the corticospinal fibers, the most frequently reported stimulation-related side effects in the GPi are contralateral contractions of tongue, throat, face, or limbs, as well as dysarthria, gagging, and facial tightness. A subjective tingling sensation may occur before any visible muscle contraction, providing a warning signal. Flashing lights and phosphenes can be caused when stimulating the most ventral electrodes, which are placed near the optic tract. As noted for the other DBS targets, reducing stimulation amplitude or switching to a different active contact normally resolves these problems.

Mechanisms of action

The clinical outcomes of DBS have been much more clearly elucidated than the mechanisms whereby it works. Several theories have tried to explain the neurophysiology underlying the success of stimulation. It is currently speculated that DBS modulates neural activity on a much larger scale than can be explained by excitation or inhibition at the cellular level. However, we have yet to arrive at an unequivocal theory encompassing the various clinical and experimental findings associated with DBS of the basal ganglia. A detailed discussion of the theories related to DBS mechanisms of action is probably beyond the scope of this chapter, but interested readers can refer to published reviews.[23] Further research using in vivo recordings and computer modeling is greatly needed in order to elucidate DBS mechanisms of action and possibly improve our understanding of PD pathophysiology.

References

1. Okun MS, Tagliati M, Pourfar M, et al. Management of referred DBS failures: a retrospective analysis from two movement disorders centers. *Arch Neurol.* 2005;62:1250–1255.

2. Lang AE, Houeto JL, Krack P, et al. Deep brain stimulation: preoperative issues. *Mov Disord*. 2006;21(suppl 14):S171–S196.

3. Pillon B. Neuropsychological assessment for management of patients with deep brain stimulation. *Mov Disord*. 2002;17(suppl 3):S116–S122.

4. Shils J, Tagliati M, Alterman R. Neurophysiological monitoring during neuro-surgery for movement disorders. In: Deletis V, Shils J, eds. *Neurophysiology in Neurosurgery*. San Diego: Academic Press; 2002:393–436.

5. Holloway KL, Gaede SE, Starr PA, et al. Frameless stereotaxy using bone fiducial markers for deep brain stimulation. *J Neurosurg*. 2005;103:404–413.

6. Moro E, Esselink RJ, Xie J, et al. The impact on Parkinson's disease of electrical parameter settings in STN stimulation. *Neurology*. 2002;59:706–713.

7. Krack P, Fraix V, Mendes A, et al. Postoperative management of subtha-lamic nucleus stimulation for Parkinson's disease. *Mov Disord*. 2002;17(suppl 3):S188–S197.

8. Alterman RL, Shils JL, Gudesblatt M, Tagliati M. Immediate and sustained relief of levodopa-induced dyskinesias after dorsal relocation of a deep brain stimula-tion lead. Case report. *Neurosurg Focus*. 2004;17:E6.

9. The Deep-Brain Stimulation for Parkinson's Disease Study Group. Deep-brain stimulation of the subthalamic nucleus or the pars interna of the globus pallidus in Parkinson's disease. *N Engl J Med*. 2001;345:956–963.

10. Limousin P, Speelman JD, Gielen F, et al. Multicentre European study of thalamic stimulation in Parkinsonian and essential tremor. *J Neurol Neurosurg Psychiatry*. 1999;66:289–296.

11. Pahwa R, Lyons KE, Wilkinson SB, et al. Long term evaluation of deep brain stimulation of the thalamus. *J Neurosurg*. 2006;104:506–512.

12. Deuschl G, Schade-Britten C, Krack P, et al. A randomized trial of deep-brain stimulation for Parkinson's disease. *N Engl J Med*. 2006;355:896–908.

13. Kleiner-Fisman G, Herzog J, Fisman D, et al. Subthalamic nucleus deep brain stimulation: summary and meta-analysis of outcomes. *Mov Disord*. 2006;21(suppl 14):S290–S304.

14. Ghika J, Villemure JG, Fankhauser H, et al. Efficiency and safety of bilateral contemporaneous pallidal stimulation (deep brain stimulation) in levodopa-responsive patients with Parkinson's disease with severe motor fluctuations: a 2 year follow-up review. *J Neurosurg*. 1998;89:713–718.

15. Volkmann J, Allert N, Voges J, Sturm V, Schnitzler A, Freund HJ. Long-term results of bilateral pallidal stimulation in Parkinson's disease. *Ann Neurol*. 2004;55:871–875.

16. Lyons KE, Wilkinson SB, Troster AI, Pahwa R. Long-term efficacy of globus pallidus stimulation for the treatment of Parkinson's disease. *Stereotact Funct Neurosurg*. 2002;79:214–220.

17. Rezai AR, Kopell BH, Gross RE, et al. Deep brain stimulation for Parkinson's disease: surgical issues. *Mov Disord*. 2006;21(suppl 14):S197–S218.

18. Schuurman PR, Bosch DA, Bossuyt PM, et al. A comparison of continuous tha-lamic stimulation and thalamotomy for suppression of severe tremor. *N Engl J Med*. 2000;342:461–468.

19. Shivitz N, Koop MM, Fahimi J, Heit G, Bronte-Stewart HM. Bilateral subtha-lamic nucleus deep brain stimulation improves certain aspects of postural control in Parkinson's disease, whereas medication does not. *Mov Disord*. 2006;21:1088–1097.

20. Voon V, Kubu C, Krack P, Houeto JL, Troster AI. Deep brain stimulation: neuropsychological and neuropsychiatric issues. *Mov Disord.* 2006;21 (suppl 14):S305–S327.

21. Temel Y, Kessels A, Tan S, Topdag A, Boon P, Visser-Vandewalle V. Behavioural changes after bilateral subthalamic stimulation in advanced Parkinson disease: a systematic review. *Parkinsonism Relat Disord.* 2006;12:265–272.

22. Bejjani BP, Damier P, Arnulf I, et al. Transient acute depression induced by high-frequency deep-brain stimulation. *N Engl J Med.* 1999;340:1476–1480.

23. Montgomery EB Jr, Gale JT. Mechanisms of action of deep brain stimulation (DBS). *Neurosci Biobehav Rev.* 2007 [Epub ahead of print].

Chapter 10

Nonpharmacological management of Parkinson's disease

Aleksandar Videnovic

Parkinson's disease (PD) is a progressive neurodegenerative disorder associated with significant disability in both motor and nonmotor functional domains. Pharmacological and surgical treatments have significantly improved the symptomatic burden of PD. However, due to the progressive nature of PD, these therapies often become ineffective with time, and may cause intolerable adverse events. There is therefore a tremendous need to optimize the utilization of nonpharmacological rehabilitative therapies with the aim of improving function and quality of life in the PD population. This chapter summarizes the role of nonpharmacological therapies in the management of PD patients.

Physical therapy

The aim of physical therapy (PT) in PD is to optimize functional ability and reduce secondary complications through movement rehabilitation within a context of education and support. It is estimated that up to 60% of PD patients are referred to a physiotherapist at some point during their disease.[1]

The PT assessment begins with a comprehensive history that should focus on the current functional level. In addition to motor symptoms, other comorbidities, such as depression, dementia, visual and hearing impairments, and cardiovascular and pulmonary limitations, need to be identified. A careful review of medications is obligatory. A collateral history obtained from caregivers and family members may provide invaluable additional information. Physical examination is focused on range of motion; gross muscle strength; resistance to passive movement; timed performance of activities; and tests of balance, motor planning, and learning ability. Based on the initial findings, a problem list is created, and short- and long-term treatment goals are identified. The goals and approaches of PT will vary across the spectrum of PD. In early de novo patients, the major objective of PT intervention is teaching the role of exercise in a healthy lifestyle. With the progression of disability, baseline limitations and impairments are assessed, and core PT strategies for the optimization of locomotion and physical activity are applied. In advanced disease, the objective is to teach patients and caregivers compensatory strategies in order to achieve functional goals, such as getting out of bed or finishing a meal, and to modify activities of daily living (ADL) according to the disability level. It is crucial to establish realistic expectations before PT commences.

Rigidity, one of the distinctive characteristics of PD, often indirectly leads to musculoskeletal and respiratory impairments. PT should focus on reduction of rigidity through the use of regular, frequent stretching and range-of-motion exercises. Patients are instructed to focus on the rotation at major joints, particularly shoulders, as these are prone to pain and stiffness. An early goal of PT is to restore normal alignment, mobility, and flexibility of the neck and trunk, since the joint mobility in these areas becomes compromised early in PD. This will also improve abnormal posture. Core muscle strengthening of the abdominal, paraspinal, and pelvic girdle musculature is crucial to improvement of mobility and transfers. A structured aerobic exercise program is designed to address low endurance, a common complaint among PD patients. Resistive exercises should be used cautiously since PD patients have difficulty with the initiation and maintenance of muscle contraction. Walking is probably the best and safest exercise for most patients. Swimming is great for muscle tone and endurance. Group exercises that involve the patient's spouse or caregiver, or even other patients, may enhance socialization and compliance.[2]

Gait dysfunction becomes one of the major challenges with the progression of PD. While there are no validated guidelines for specific gait training in PD, a number of strategies have been shown to be effective. External visual, auditory, or proprioceptive cues can facilitate continuous movements. Cognitive strategies, such as sequencing of functional activities (getting out of bed, getting dressed, etc.) may further help to overcome motor planning and programming deficits. Patients should be urged to take larger steps and reminded to swing their arms. Freezing of gait is one of the most disturbing symptoms of PD. "Start hesitation" and freezing on turning are the most common types of freezing. Various motor and sensory tricks can be employed to overcome freezing of gait. The most commonly used techniques are auditory and verbal stimuli, such as giving marching commands or using rhythmic cues generated by a metronome, sometimes embedded in music. Stride length and freezing may further be improved by placing lines on the floor and instructing patients to step over them.

Postural instability is the hallmark of advanced PD. Pharmacological treatments are of limited value in correcting this symptom. PT can offer compensatory strategies and improve ambulation safety. There are no established guidelines on the use of assistive devices for gait impairment in PD. Impaired coordination of upper and lower extremities poses challenges to the use of a cane or walker. Patients will often drag a cane or carry a walker, which increases the risk of falling. Therefore, the need for an assistive device should be assessed by a physiotherapist, and education about its appropriate use should be provided to the patient. Home PT is indicated when travel is difficult or when the home environment requires modification.

Breathing exercises and chest expansion strategies become important in advanced stages of the disease when vital capacity diminishes, leading to an increased risk of aspiration. These exercises can provide added benefit when combined with speech therapy.

Based on recently published evidence-based recommendations, the core areas for PT in PD include transfers, posture, reaching and grasping, balance, gait, and physical activity.[3] Key recommendations are the application of cueing strategies to improve gait, cognitive movement strategies to improve transfers, and specific exercises to improve balance and training of joint mobility and muscle power. Despite a considerable body of literature, systematic reviews of published clinical trials found little or no evidence to support or refute the efficacy of PT in PD.[4,5] The main shortcomings of published studies are methodological flaws, small number of patients, and large differences in the PT intervention. Large and well-designed randomized controlled trials of effectiveness of PT in PD are needed.

Occupational therapy

The role of occupational therapy (OT) in early PD is to enable patients to maintain their usual level of self-care, work, and leisure activities for as long as possible. With disease progression, OT becomes focused on the development of modified activities and identification of new roles for the patient. These efforts are ultimately directed to minimize disability and improve quality of life. It is estimated that only 13% to 25% of PD patients are assessed by an occupational therapist during their disease.[6] Patients are usually referred for OT later in the course of disease, at the point when many limitations in ADL or work have already emerged.

The initial step in OT is to obtain a comprehensive history that assesses the patient's ability to perform specific tasks and ADL. This initial assessment should be followed with a detailed OT evaluation focusing on strength, coordination, and range of motion. The patient's ability to perform work-specific activities and ADL should be tested by having them simulate various tasks. Improvements achieved with PT and OT complement each other, so both therapies should be instituted simultaneously.

ADL may have to be modified and broken down into several components. There are many assistive devices and types of equipment that can be used to enhance performance of everyday tasks. Examples include grab rails, spill-proof cups, nonslip trays and plates, jar openers, electric toothbrushes, and clothing with Velcro fastenings. Firm mattresses, nonslip sheets, and loose bed covers may help with changing position overnight. Lift chairs may facilitate transfers. On-site home visits improve safety by identifying possible hazards and tailoring the home environment to the patient's needs. Bathtubs may have to be replaced with showers, and toilets may need to be elevated. Rugs should be removed or backed with adhesive material to keep them from slipping. Occupational limitations may necessitate a change in the patient's employment.

Education of the patient as well as of family members and caregivers is a crucial component throughout the OT process. OT should be offered not only to patients with advanced disease but also to patients with early disease, who, despite the lack of significant motor impairment, often suffer the emotional and psychological stigma of PD that can negatively affect their work and ADL.

Clinical experience suggests that OT may provide valuable benefits to PD patients, although a recent systematic review by The Cochrane Collaboration found insufficient evidence to support its efficacy in PD.[6] Evidence-based medicine research of OT in PD is challenged by methodological issues, including open-label designs, small number of patients, and variations in intervention paradigms and outcome measures. Deane et al.[7,8] recently published a consensus on standard OT in PD. Further studies employing innovative designs, larger numbers of patients, carefully defined therapeutic protocols, and outcome measures are needed for an accurate estimate of benefit achieved with OT in PD.

Speech and swallowing therapies

Speech therapy

Speech disorders affect almost every PD patient as the disease progresses. Reduced voice volume (hypophonia) may be one of the presenting symptoms of PD. Other speech disturbances include a breathy, hoarse voice quality (dysphonia), imprecise articulation, monotony of pitch and volume (dysprosody), and variations in speed that result in rushed, hesitant, or stuttered speech. The spectrum of speech disturbances in PD is referred to as hypokinetic dysarthria.

Improvements in speech quality with pharmacological treatments are often very limited, and surgical interventions are usually associated with worsening of speech intelligibility. In these circumstances the benefits of speech and language therapy should be maximized. Despite the very common occurrence of speech dysfunction in PD, reportedly only up to 20% of PD patients are seen by a speech and language therapist.[9] Speech therapy in PD incorporates traditional approaches as well as newer methods such as the Lee Silverman voice treatment (LSVT) program.

Traditional speech therapy utilizes various breathing and prosodic exercises to improve articulation precision, rate, vocal loudness, and pitch. Delayed auditory feedback may improve speech intelligibility and loudness. With these traditional methods, achieved improvements are modest and short-lived. Prosthetic and augmentative devices, such as voice amplifiers, have been studied in a small number of PD patients, and their use remains limited.

The LSVT program, named for one of the first patients treated with this method, was developed by Ramig and Mead in the early 1980s.[10] The treatment focuses on voice therapy rather than speech therapy. This is intensive, 16-session treatment (4 times a week for 1 month) designed to elicit a louder voice with good quality. An increased vocal cord adduction seems to be a key element in treatment success. During treatment sessions patients are required to speak loudly. Several exercises targeting duration, constant loudness, and voice steadiness are implemented. The high-effort level of speech production that is established during the treatment sessions is crucial for a successful transition to the outside environment. Other keys to success with LSVT are habituation and calibration of patients to the new phonatory effort level. During these processes patients become comfortable with a louder voice, which prevents them from losing achieved benefits. The treatment is terminated once the patient has demonstrated the ability to speak with increased loudness 85% of the time in conversational speech in the treatment facility and 70% of the time outside of the treatment facility. Patients are encouraged to continue with exercises at home after the treatment is completed. Patients with mild to moderate PD receive the greatest benefit, which emphasizes the need for early administration of the treatment. Patients with advanced PD coexistent with depression and dementia do not achieve great improvement with the treatment. Significant improvements in duration of phonation, phonation range, and perceptual aspects of speech such as intelligibility and loudness have been documented after the treatment, with long-term benefits persisting up to 6 to 12 months.[11] In addition to improvements of vocal characteristics and articulation, functional imaging using positron emission tomography have demonstrated neural plasticity changes in speech brain areas after the treatment.[12] The beneficial effects of the LSVT on tongue strength and motility, swallowing, and facial expression have also been documented.

Despite positive experiences with speech intervention in the PD population, several recent evidence-based medicine reviews found insufficient evidence to support or refute the efficacy of speech therapy for hypokinetic dysarthria in PD.[6,9] Larger randomized, controlled trials with carefully selected outcome measures and longer follow-up are needed.

Swallowing therapy

Swallowing disorders are common among PD patients, especially with the progression of the disease. Abnormalities in all phases of swallowing (oral preparatory, oral, pharyngeal, and esophageal) have been documented.[13] Reduction in tongue strength and control with impaired ability to initiate swallowing reflex are common abnormalities in the oral phase. The pharyngeal phase is usually compromised by food residues and prolonged transit time. Slow and incomplete laryngeal closure is yet another deficit. These impairments collectively contribute to choking, reduced ability to take oral medications, reduced caloric intake, and risks for aspiration. This mandates timely recognition and appropriate assessment and treatment of dysphagia in the PD population.

The management of dysphagia requires a team effort, and a speech-language pathologist represents the core of this team. The initial step is to regularly inquire about swallowing difficulties during clinic visits.

The threshold for a formal swallow evaluation should be low. An initial "bedside" evaluation is usually followed by a video swallowing assessment. Recommendations about diet changes, need for assistive devices to facilitate eating, or modifications in body positioning during meals are based on the assessment's outcome. Literature on therapeutic interventions for swallowing dysfunction in PD is sparse. Traditional therapy approaches utilize various oral exercises to improve muscle strength and coordination. Consultation with a nutritionist ensures the adequacy of the caloric intake when diet modifications are needed. Several behavioral modifications, such as alternating sips of liquid with food or a multiple-swallow technique, may further improve swallowing. The "chin-tuck" posture, during which a patient holds the chin down, close to the chest, may improve airway closure during swallowing. If these efforts do not improve swallowing and the patient develops significant aspiration, weight loss, or dehydration, alternatives to oral feeding should be explored. This decision is always based on the comprehensive assessment of the patient's physical condition, cognitive performance, living arrangements, and personal wishes.

Complementary and alternative medicine

Complementary and alternative medicine (CAM) incorporates a group of diverse medical health-care systems, practices, and products that are not presently considered to be part of conventional medicine. Treatment modalities of CAM can be broadly categorized into herbal/nutritional, mind-body, body-based, and energetic. Although CAM is increasingly utilized by the general population, existing research in this area among the PD population is limited by the paucity of well-designed studies. However, it is estimated that up to 40% of PD patients use at least one form of CAM, most commonly in conjunction with conventional therapies for PD.[14]

Acupuncture

Acupuncture has been used as a part of traditional Chinese medicine for centuries and is now one of the most commonly used treatment modalities of CAM among PD patients.[14] Although only a few studies have assessed the role of acupuncture in PD, it seems to be safe and well tolerated. Most patients report subjective improvement after acupuncture. The effects of acupuncture on motor symptoms of PD are controversial; while some authors document mild improvements, others report worsening of motor scores.[15,16] Eng et al.[15] found significant improvement in depressive symptoms among PD patients treated with Chinese energy massage and acupuncture over 6 months. Limitations of available published studies include lack of a control group, differences in acupuncture methods used, variable duration of intervention, and potential placebo effect. Recently, the electro-acupuncture method, which involves the placement of needles subcutaneously over nonacupuncture points in control subjects, has been used in an attempt to address the issue of controls in acupuncture interventions in PD.[17] These techniques require further validation studies. Similar to other modalities of CAM, well-designed, randomized, controlled trials are needed in order to establish the role of acupuncture in patients with PD.

Massage

Massage has been used in the ancient Indian medicine system of ayurveda in the treatment of PD, which was known as *kampavata*. Massage therapy is utilized by about 10% of PD patients.[14] Improvements in self-confidence, well-being, walking, and ADL have been documented in PD patients after massage treatments.[18] Rigidity and tremors may also improve following massage. These benefits are based on clinical observations, because this treatment can not be tested using a double-blind approach. It has been suggested that massage may stimulate the release of dopamine, endorphins, and substance P, leading to relaxation of muscles and joints. The beneficial effects of massage may also be related to alleviation of anxiety.

Exercise

Positive impacts of physical exercise on physiological and psychological well-being have been well established in the general population. Several studies have confirmed these benefits in the PD population.[19] Animal studies utilizing treadmill exercise documented changes in dopaminergic neurotransmission associated with improvements in motor performance.[20] Physical exercise is associated with lower mortality in the PD population,[21] and may have protective effects on the risk for developing PD. In addition to improvements in PD-specific motor disability, exercise increases perceived functional independence and quality of life.[22] Patients should be advised during the early stages of the disease to develop a regular exercise program. Regular adherence to physical exercise is crucial, since the benefits may wear off after several months of inactivity. Available exercises are numerous and patients should be encouraged to select a type they will enjoy. Exercises that emphasize balance and core strengthening, such as Pilates, yoga, and tai chi, may be excellent choices for this population.

Herbal medicines and nutritional supplements

Herbal medicines are widely used but very poorly studied among PD patients. Oxidative stress has been implicated in the pathogenesis of PD, providing a rationale for the use of selected nutritional supplements as adjuncts to conventional treatments in PD. The most commonly used supplements are vitamins E and C, coenzyme Q10, calcium, glutathione, and Ensure. Supplement use is often initiated without a consultation by a treating physician. Despite the frequent supplement use, PD patients often lack knowledge about possible adverse effects or drug interactions. Physicians therefore must inquire about the use of supplements and provide appropriate counseling. Coenzyme Q10 has been shown to be safe and potentially slows the progression of PD disability, but additional data are necessary, and a large pivotal study is planned. Vitamin E did not demonstrate efficacy as a neuroprotective agent in a large placebo-controlled clinical trial. Glutathione improved disability in a small cohort of PD patients, but the effects were very small and controls were not included.

A recent systematic review of the efficacy and safety of herbal medicines for PD found insufficient evidence to recommend their use.[23]

In summary, CAM is being used more often by patients with PD. Lack of systematic studies of various CAM modalities precludes evidence-based medicine recommendations with regard to its efficacy and safety. Systematic, well-designed studies of alternative treatment modalities in PD are needed to overcome these uncertainties.

References

1. Keus SH, Bloem BR, Verbaan D, et al. Physiotherapy in Parkinson's disease: utilisation and patient satisfaction. *J Neurol.* 2004;251(6):680–687.

2. Gauthier L, Dalziel S, Gauthier S. The benefits of group occupational therapy for patients with Parkinson's disease. *Am J Occup Ther.* 1987;41(6):360–365.

3. Keus SH, Bloem BR, Hendriks EJ, Bredero-Cohen AB, Munneke M. Evidence-based analysis of physical therapy in Parkinson's disease with recommendations for practice and research. *Mov Disord.* 2007;22(4):451–460; quiz 600.

4. Deane KH, Jones D, Playford ED, Ben-Shlomo Y, Clarke CE. Physiotherapy for patients with Parkinson's Disease: a comparison of techniques. *Cochrane Database Syst Rev.* 2001;(3):CD002817.

5. Gage H, Storey L. Rehabilitation for Parkinson's disease: a systematic review of available evidence. *Clin Rehabil.* 2004;18(5):463–482.

6. Deane KH, Ellis-Hill C, Playford ED, Ben-Shlomo Y, Clarke CE. Occupational therapy for patients with Parkinson's disease. *Cochrane Database Syst Rev.* 2001;(3):CD002813.

7. Deane KH, Ellis-Hill C, Dekker K, Davies P, Clarke CE. A survey of current occupational therapy practice for Parkinson's disease in the United Kingdom. *British Journal of Occupational Therapy.* 2003;66(5):193–200.

8. Deane KH, Ellis-Hill C, Dekker K, Davies P, Clarke CE. A Delphi survey of best practice occupational therapy for Parkinson's disease in the United Kingdom. *British Journal of Occupational Therapy.* 2003;66(6):247–254.

9. Deane KH, Whurr R, Playford ED, Ben-Shlomo Y, Clarke CE. A comparison of speech and language therapy techniques for dysarthria in Parkinson's disease. *Cochrane Database Syst Rev.* 2001;(2):CD002814.

10. Ramig LO, Countryman S, O'Brien C, Hoehn M, Thompson L. Intensive speech treatment for patients with Parkinson's disease: short- and long-term comparison of two techniques. *Neurology.* 1996;47(6):1496–1504.

11. Sapir S, Ramig LO, Hoyt P, Countryman S, O'Brien C, Hoehn M. Speech loudness and quality 12 months after intensive voice treatment (LSVT) for Parkinson's disease: a comparison with an alternative speech treatment. *Folia Phoniatr Logop.* 2002;54(6):296–303.

12. Liotti M, Ramig LO, Vogel D, et al. Hypophonia in Parkinson's disease: neural correlates of voice treatment revealed by PET. *Neurology.* 2003;60(3):432–440.

13. Johnston BT, Li Q, Castell JA, Castell DO. Swallowing and esophageal function in Parkinson's disease. *Am J Gastroenterol.* 1995;90(10):1741–1746.

14. Rajendran PR, Thompson RE, Reich SG. The use of alternative therapies by patients with Parkinson's disease. *Neurology.* 2001;57(5):790–794.

15. Eng ML, Lyons KE, Greene MS, Pahwa R. Open-label trial regarding the use of acupuncture and yin tui na in Parkinson's disease outpatients: a pilot

study on efficacy, tolerability, and quality of life. *J Altern Complement Med.* 2006;12(4):395–399.

16. Shulman LM, Wen X, Weiner WJ, et al. Acupuncture therapy for the symptoms of Parkinson's disease. *Mov Disord.* 2002;17(4):799–802.

17. Cristian A, Katz M, Cutrone E, Walker RH. Evaluation of acupuncture in the treatment of Parkinson's disease: a double-blind pilot study. *Mov Disord.* 2005;20(9):1185–1188.

18. Paterson C, Allen JA, Browning M, Barlow G, Ewings P. A pilot study of therapeutic massage for people with Parkinson's disease: the added value of user involvement. *Complement Ther Clin Pract.* 2005;11(3):161–171.

19. Crizzle AM, Newhouse IJ. Is physical exercise beneficial for persons with Parkinson's disease? *Clin J Sport Med.* 2006;16(5):422–425.

20. Petzinger GM, Walsh JP, Akopian G, et al. Effects of treadmill exercise on dopaminergic transmission in the 1-methyl-4-phenyl-1,2,3,6-tetrahydropyridine-lesioned mouse model of basal ganglia injury. *J Neurosci.* 2007;27(20):5291–5300.

21. Kuroda K, Tatara K, Takatorige T, Shinsho F. Effect of physical exercise on mortality in patients with Parkinson's disease. *Acta Neurol Scand.* 1992;86(1):55–59.

22. Sasco AJ, Paffenbarger RS Jr, Gendre I, Wing AL. The role of physical exercise in the occurrence of Parkinson's disease. *Arch Neurol.* 1992;49(4):360–365.

23. Chung V, Liu L, Bian Z, et al. Efficacy and safety of herbal medicines for idiopathic Parkinson's disease: a systematic review. *Mov Disord.* 2006;21(10):1709–1715.

Index